A HEALTHY

A HEALTHY 10!

A Reference Guide for Gymnasts
& Other Athletes

by

Jack E. Jensen, MD
Leslie Spencer, LAT
Linda Angela Day

Houston, 1992

For information about permission to reproduce selections from this book, write to Jack E. Jensen, MD, Athletic Orthopedics & Knee Center, 9180 Old Katy Road, Suite 200, Houston, Texas 77055

Library of Congress Cataloging in Publication Data

Jensen, Jack E.
    A Healthy 10! : a gymnast's personal reference guide /
        Jack E. Jensen

        p. cm.

    Includes index.
    ISBN 0-9633870.8.1 (paperback)
    1. Sports Health
1.   Title.
92.097010 CIP

Printed in the United States of America

Book Design: Tompkins & Tompkins

CONTENTS

v

CONTENTS

CONTENTS

CONTENTS

CONTENTS

CONTENTS

DEDICATION

This book is dedicated to Allison, Kristin, Justin and the athletes I have treated.

JJ, *Fall 1992*

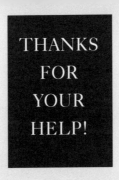

THANKS FOR YOUR HELP!

I want to express gratitude to all the people who have done so much to help create this book.

Like Judith McClain, who managed the infinite details involved in putting it all together. It's hard to imagine having done it without her. And Teresa Zavala, who was always available for *whatever* needed to be done. (It didn't hurt that Teresa's also an ex-gymnast!)

My sincere appreciation goes to Bela and Martha Karolyi for their confidence in me, allowing me the incredible experience of being their team physician.

Coauthors Linda and Leslie made it all possible by taking my thoughts and ideas and turning them into this book!

Equal thanks goes to my wife Allison, who supported me in her multiple roles as wife, mother and dietitian. In fact, she contributed significantly to the development of the nutrition chapter.

And finally, for visually capturing the spirit of this book, I thank my graphic design firm, Tompkins & Tompkins.

Jack E. Jensen, MD FACSM
Fall 1992

Introduction

What would you like from this book? Are you a gymnast who wants information to help you excel? Are you a parent who wants your child to get everything from the sport except a damaged body? Are you a coach who wants to achieve top conditioning, safely? Perhaps you're starting a gymnastics program and need some medical advice. Or perhaps you just want a handy guide for gymnastics medical questions.

Maybe you're not a gymnast at all, but only want easy-to-understand sports medicine information.

If any of this fits, we think you've come to the right place. Although we direct and dedicate this book to gymnasts, we're writing for all of you.

And who are "we?" Well. . .

■ Jack E. Jensen, MD, is a Fellow and Clinical Board Member of the Texas chapter of the American College of Sports Medicine and a Clinical Assistant Professor at the University of Texas Medical School in Houston. He's had years of experience treating gymnasts and other athletes—from the very young to the Olympic elite, male and female. Jack is the medical mind and the man with the vision to put this book together.

■ Leslie Spencer is Jack's Licensed Athletic Trainer (LAT) who has worked extensively with both young and Olympic gymnasts. Leslie has contributed many of the exercises and much of the other training expertise.

■ Linda Day is the award-winning writer who makes the knowledge and experience of Jack and Leslie easy to understand and fun to read. With an advanced degree in biochemistry and many years as a dedicated skier, kayaker, Jazzerciser and all-round fitness aficionado, Linda has a keen interest in sports medicine.

xiv

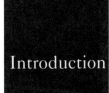

Introduction

You'll meet all of us in the pages of this book, often by name. Why are we writing this book? We know it's possible to get to "the perfect 10"—but it's most important to do it in a safe, healthy way.

According to the statistics, injury rates tend to go up as you get more competitive. The injury rate for non-competitive gymnasts is much lower (0.04 percent to 0.07 percent) than for beginning competitors (0.7 percent). For advanced gymnasts, the rate goes up to 5.3 percent. (Don't panic—remember, this is still only about one in 20.)

The injury rate is higher for all elite athletes because they work so much harder and spend so much more time at it. A close look reveals that injury rates stay lower when sports are carefully supervised by coaches and trainers who promote training without straining. We write this book to help their efforts. We want gymnasts and parents to have the information they need about the body, nutrition, training, injuries and prevention.

That's what this book is about—how best to fulfill your own potential. And maybe get a perfect *healthy* 10 along the way.

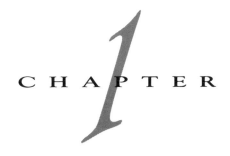

C H A P T E R

The Medical
Team

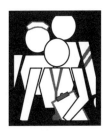

When you get involved with a gymnastics team, you'll find there are important team members who never swing from the high bar or manage even the simplest round-off. These are the people whose job it is to keep you healthy and help you recover quickly from injuries. For simplicity, we'll call them the medical team, although many of them aren't doctors.

In just about all areas of life, it helps to have the right tool: It's hard to drive a nail with a screwdriver or turn a screw with a wrench. The different members of the medical team are like that, too—each person is best suited to help you in a particular way. The more you know about the way they can (and can't) help, the better off you'll be.

CALLING ALL DOCTORS

Did you know that the first name for doctors was *gymnastes*? These were Greeks who specialized in the training of Olympic athletes. Herodicus (born about 400 BC) was one of the most famous. He wrote about diet, exercise and physical rehabilitation, key concerns of ours today. His student Hippocrates even prescribed exercise as a remedy for mental illness. Hippocrates also wrote the Hippocratic Oath, which binds all physicians practicing today.

Of course nowadays physicians worry about much more than exercise. And there is more than one kind of doctor. In gymnastics, you may meet four: medical doctors, osteopaths, chiropractors, and podiatrists.

The Medical Doctor (M.D.)

Of all the doctors, the M.D. has the most schooling, including a minimum of four years of college, four years of medical school and one year of internship. As an intern, the doctor spends an average of 25 hours a day or more working in a hospital and attending patients with all kinds of different problems. At the end of the internship, the doctor is officially a general practitioner who can see patients and prescribe medications.

Most doctors go beyond internship to become specialists: This requires a residency, which can last anywhere from one to five years. Like interns, residents work in hospitals, but they are higher up the totem pole and so they spend something less than 25 hours a day on call. Nearly all of their time is spent learning more about one particular field of medicine.

In the United States and Canada, there are currently 23 distinct specialties, each with its own rule-making body, called a *board*. When a doctor is "board certified" in a particular specialty, he or she has passed extensive tests given by that Board. A general surgeon may carry out plastic surgery procedures, but may not have board certification. If you want to make sure you are choosing a physician with complete training in a specialty, look for American board certification.

We mention "American" board certification because many upstart boards have appeared in recent years. Some of these new boards have very minimal requirements for membership, which effectively allows doctors with questionable qualifications to claim "board" certification. To make sure you are getting the genuine article, look for certification by the American Board of whatever-it-is.

Orthopedics and Sports Medicine

Next to your family doctor, these are the doctors you may see the most as a gymnast:

Orthopedics

Orthopedists (sometimes referred to by the space-age jargon of "orthopods") take care of diseases and problems relating to bones, joints and muscles. The specialty had its beginnings in treating childhood deformities—*orthopedics* literally means *straight child;* today these doctors help people of all ages.

Orthopedic work can involve surgery—repairing injured knees and shoulders and replacing joints—but more often it does not. The orthopedist spends the most time in non-surgical medicine, prescribing rehabilitation techniques. As an orthopedist, Jack spends much more time devising exercise programs than he does cutting and sewing.

Sports Medicine

Sports medicine is a subspecialty of orthopedics, although it is really so encompassing that no one person can know it all. Everyone we talk about in this chapter can be part of a sports medicine team. And doctors who you might think would have nothing to do with sports medicine can be very involved. For example, a pulmonary specialist (a sub-specialty of internal medicine) might be an expert in exercise-induced asthma, which is sports medicine! Another example is the internist who directs a rehabilitation program following mononucleosis.

As it relates to orthopedics, sports medicine deals with preventing and treating injuries that result from sports. This is Dr. Jensen's discipline.

To become trained in sports medicine, an orthopedist must spend from several months to a year in a fellowship program following residency. The sports medicine doctor may have a total of ten years of medical training.

Sports medicine requires quite a bit of specialized knowledge, because athletes injure themselves in so many ways, and the nature of the injury depends on the sport in which it occurred. Injuries tend to occur wherever a sport requires repetitive use. Terms like "tennis elbow," "pitcher's elbow," "swimmer's shoulder" and, alas, "gymnast's wrist" illustrate the point.

Sometimes odd body parts can play an unexpected key role. For example, a toe injury ended Dizzy Dean's pitching career! The toe pain altered his pitching motion, which in turn stressed his arm enough to produce the injury that forced him to stop pitching.

If you pick a sports medicine doctor, be careful to make sure it is someone who really understands gymnastics and who has specialized training or expertise in sports medicine. Just because someone says in the phone book that they are a sports medicine doctor does not mean that's what they do. Check whether the doctor is board-certified. It's okay to ask for references, to ask what percentage of their practice relates to sports injuries, and to ask how many gymnasts they see in their practice. A reputable doctor won't be offended if you ask pointed questions about qualifications. If the doctor gets huffy about it, go elsewhere.

Physical Medicine and Rehabilitation

Doctors trained in this specialty are called "physiatrists," a word that sounds like *psychiatrist* but isn't. Physiatrists work to rehabilitate patients after injuries or illnesses, and they specialize in exercise programs and the use of whirlpool, electrical stimulation, and other rehabilitative techniques. They combine a knowledge of medicine with expertise in athletic training and physical therapy (see following) and often work closely with an orthopedist as part of a sports medicine team.

Other Medical Specialties

In addition to the doctors involved most directly with your sport, you may also become familiar with other specialties:

Family practice

In the old days, many family doctors were simple general practitioners. Nowadays, most family doctors have specialized in Family Practice. Family practitioners treat mostly teenagers and adults, and some younger folks.

Internal medicine

The internist is concerned about the diagnosis and treatment of adults with diseases of the internal organs. Many internists are primary-care physicians; they have a direct relationship with patients on a long-term basis. Generally, it's an internist (or a family practitioner) who will refer you to another specialist if you need one.

There are nine subspecialties in internal medicine that focus on specific organs, but we'll spare you the details.

Pediatrics

Pediatrics has the same focus as internal medicine, except it deals with babies and children. Pediatrics, too, has subspecialties, including a relatively new one, adolescent medicine.

Allergy and immunology

These specialists deal with various allergies (including food allergies), asthma and other hypersensitivity disorders.

The Doctor of Osteopathy (D.O.)

Osteopathy began in 1892 with a school founded by Andrew Taylor Still, who felt that the main obstacle to good

health was faulty alignment of the bones. Still lived at a
Shawnee Indian mission in Kansas in 1853, and some think that
his hands-on approach to healing came from the Indians.

Originally, osteopaths did not do surgery or prescribe
medicine, but today osteopathic schools offer courses very
similar to those taught in medical schools. Osteopaths specialize
in manipulating areas of the body to restore correct alignment of
bones and muscles and they may also prescribe drugs and carry
out surgery.

To become an osteopath requires two years of college,
four years of study at an accredited osteopathic school, and an
internship. Osteopaths may also specialize by taking graduate
courses in surgery, pediatrics and internal medicine, and they
may also take medical residencies.

There are about three-hundred osteopathic hospitals
and numerous clinics in the United States today.

The Doctor of Chiropractic (D.C.)

Chiropractic was instigated by Daniel David Palmer
(1845-1913), an Iowa grocer who coined the term from the
Greek words meaning "practice by hand." Today there are
about fifteen accredited chiropractic colleges in the United
States and Canada. For admission, the applicant must have a
high-school diploma and often at least two years of college. The
four years of chiropractic training include courses on anatomy,
chemistry, neurology, physiology, x-ray diagnosis and other
subjects. Training also includes an internship period in the
school's clinics.

The American Medical Association recognized
chiropractic in 1980 and now permits medical doctors to
recommend patients to chiropractors. In addition, chiropractors
can now admit patients to hospitals and treat them there.

Chiropractors do not use drugs or surgery; they treat
problems by manipulating the spine, joints and muscles to
restore proper nerve function. The chiropractor may also use

physical therapy techniques (ultrasound, massage, etc.) and include exercise and diet recommendations as part of the treatment.

The Doctor of Podiatric Medicine (D.P.M.)

As you've seen by now, doctors spend years specializing in one thing or another. But while most doctors get quite a bit of education about the body as a whole, podiatrists specialize in feet, both medically and surgically. To be a licensed podiatrist requires four years of advanced education in a school of podiatry. Podiatrists can prescribe medicine and carry out surgery.

Some podiatrists also sub-specialize in sports medicine, working with feet, ankles and gait problems related to sports performance.

Choosing a Doctor

No one person can do it all—every member of the medical team is a valuable player. Each professional has a slightly different approach to the subject, and sometimes a chiropractor can solve a problem that stumps the medical doctors.

In general, the most qualified person to direct your medical care is the sports medicine specialist: That doctor can then direct you to the most appropriate health-care professional for specific concerns.

THE ATHLETIC TRAINER

First let's start by making a clear distinction between "personal trainer" and "athletic trainer." Nowadays, it's quite upscale to employ a personal trainer to develop your own customized fitness program. Many of these people are highly knowledgeable and can do an excellent job; others have a couple of years experience at the local "fat shop" and know close to nothing. Be aware that *anyone* can call themselves a "personal trainer."

An athletic trainer, on the other hand, has had extensive schooling: four years of college (including courses on anatomy, physiology, kinesiology, and other sports medicine topics), plus 1,800 hours of apprenticeship helping the college's athletic teams. After achieving an undergraduate degree in sports medicine, the trainer may become certified by passing an all-day exam given by the National Athletic Trainers Association. The trainer may also have to pass a state licensing exam, depending on the laws in each state.

Team trainers specialize in orthopedic and performance rehabilitation. Like the physical therapist, they have the knowledge to get muscles and joints working again after an injury, but they also know how to return athletes to a pre-injury level of conditioning and performance.

Trainers work closely with the team physician. They are the first people to see an injury because they are usually around when it happens. They decide which injuries to refer to a doctor, and they care for simple injuries that don't need a doctor's care.

Trainers do many other things for the team too. They help with pre-participation physicals and maintain medical records. They get involved with nutrition, conditioning and strengthening programs. They make sure the equipment is in good order.

With all this expertise and responsibility, the athletic trainer is an indispensable member of the team.

OTHER SUPPORT PEOPLE

The Physical Therapist

Physical therapy came into existence to rehabilitate the soldiers injured in World War I, and it gained importance during the polio epidemics that raged between the thirties and fifties. Today dozens of institutions train physical therapists, and extensive graduate education is available as well.

The job of the physical therapist is to rehabilitate various disabilities using heat, ultrasound, massage, hydrotherapy and exercise. Physical therapists overlap athletic trainers: Both carry out orthopedic rehabilitation, but the physical therapist works more with non-athletes (plus stroke victims, burn victims, etc.), and the athletic trainer specializes in sports rehabilitation.

Exercise is important in either discipline: A good physical therapist or trainer will know exactly which combinations of exercises will work best to restore function. Much of the exercise work can be done at home, where it's a lot cheaper than a rehab clinic! Several years ago, Linda had surgery for rotator-cuff repair of her shoulder, which reduced the range of motion in her arm. Then she discovered a therapist nicknamed "Magic Fingers," who put her on a strict home exercise regimen. In a relatively short time, she regained full use of her arm and built shoulder muscles that prompted her teen-age son to call her "buff."

Maybe one of the key points of this story is that you— with a little talented professional help—can sometimes be your own best therapist!

The Exercise Physiologist

Physiology is a branch of biology that deals with the functions and vital processes of living organisms. In practical terms, the physiologist is concerned about your *condition*: How's your endurance? Strength? The amount of explosive power you can produce?

Exercise physiologists can have a bachelor's degree, a master's degree or a doctorate. They specialize in the science of exercise: What is your maximum oxygen uptake? What is your percentage of body fat, and how will that impact your performance? They use special testing procedures to determine the condition of your heart, lungs and muscles, and they make recommendations about how to improve it.

Physiologists do not prescribe medicine or get involved in medical problems.

The Dietitian

First, don't confuse a dietitian with a "nutritionist." A nutritionist can be anyone who proclaims themselves to be so, regardless of training or knowledge. The friendly salesperson at the local health food store who is trying to sell you kelp for your acne (or whatever) is probably *not* a dietitian.

Dietitians must meet academic requirements set by the American Dietetics Association and must complete at least a baccalaureate degree–and possibly a masters or doctorate. They are required to have an internship or hands-on experience and must complete continuing education courses. In addition, the person may also be licensed by the state and registered by the ADA.

The dietitian has the knowledge to assess your nutritional status *and* he or she knows how to improve it.

Psychologists and Psychiatrists

A psychiatrist is a medical doctor who has specialized by doing a residency in psychiatry. In general, psychiatry deals with the understanding and cure of mental disease.

Psychologists go to college and then take a Masters or doctor of philosophy (PhD). Most people think of psychologists as therapists who help people with problems. In fact, the field of psychology is quite broad and includes a loose alliance of scholars, scientists and practitioners concerned with all sorts of human and animal behavior.

Clinical psychologists are the people who devote most of their efforts to helping people who are disturbed, troubled or stressed.

Some clinical psychologists specialize in sports psychology, although there is no certification or licensing program for the specialty. Again, it's a good idea to ask questions: Has the psychologist written any books or articles on sports psychology? Worked with athletes on sports-related problems? Conducted seminars or workshops?

Look for someone who is not only interested in the psychology of performance, but also in how to handle stress, how to handle losing, and how to fit sports into a healthy approach to life.

Your Parents!

These are two very important members of your medical team. If you are sick or injured, they will most likely nurse you more than anyone else. So it helps to stay on good terms!

SUMMARY

A gymnastics team is a lot more than a coach and some gymnasts. We have reviewed the roles of various health professionals who may become involved with the team, but don't let it get confusing. The most qualified sports medicine professional overall is an orthopedic surgeon who has had a fellowship or extra training in sports medicine. That person should be your main contact point, especially if you have a problem. Sports medicine doctors may not be able to take care of all your problems, but they are still the most qualified people to refer you to others and to evaluate others' work.

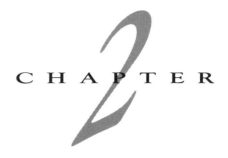

Body Basics:
The Musculoskeletal System

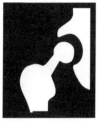

Did you know that bones are constantly changing their calcium? That some joints never move? That you'll never be able to control some muscles? That just because you can "move it" doesn't mean it "ain't broke"? No? Well, read on. This chapter will give you the basic skinny about bones, muscles, ligaments, tendons, plus the other stuff that keeps you vaulting. We'll talk about general types of injuries and conclude with some basic first aid you should know.

Really, this section should be titled the *musculo-skeleto-ligamento-tendeno-cartilagenoidal system*, because it takes more than a skeleton and some muscles to make things work. We'll start with bones.

BONES

We all know about bones, right? We see them in our chicken dinner, in the museum displays of ancient dinosaurs and in comic strips about dogs. The human body has 206 of them, and believe it or not, they are alive, living and breathing (in their own way)—not some dead chunks of calcium. They are just as much living tissue as muscle and skin, with blood vessels, nerves (yes, bones can hurt), and an active mineral life.

About 30 percent of every bone is made up of a protein called *collagen*, the same type of protein that forms your fingernails and hair. Of course, this collagen isn't stiff enough on its own. It does, however, provide the framework that supports the complicated calcium and phosphorus compounds that make bones hard and strong.

Throughout your life, calcium and phosphorus are constantly being removed and replaced in this protein framework under the control of a very complex metabolic system. You'll never have the "same old bones" because they are changing calcium like people change underwear.

The constant replacement and renewal of calcium in bones makes it possible for bones to grow and to repair themselves. It's a unique process, and nothing else in the body quite matches it.

Bone Jobs

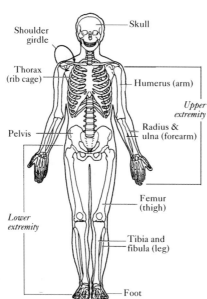

The human skeleton

Bones have two basic jobs, one of which should be obvious to you—to let you move. Nearly every life form requires something like a skeleton to enable motion: Those creatures that do without a skeleton live an unenviable slug-like existence. Even insects have skeletons, although in their case it is the crusty outside case ("exoskeleton") instead of teeny bones inside. (That's why bugs squish when you step on them and break the exoskeleton.)

The second job bones do is protect vital organs. That's

why your brain is inside your skull, your spinal cord is inside your spine, and your heart and lungs are surrounded by ribs. We could talk about bugs here, too, but perhaps enough is enough.

Bone Parts

There are two basic types of bones, designated by the intricate medical terms of "long" (like the leg bone) and "flat" (like the shoulder blade).

Long bones may have other parts: The *head* is the rounded end that allows the bone to rotate, like the head of the thigh bone where it fits into the pelvis. The *shaft* is the long midsection. *Condyles* are lumps at one or both ends of the bone where ligaments attach. And *tuberosities* and *trochanters* are bumps where tendons attach. Perhaps the most obvious tuberosity (if you're looking for an example) is the *tibial tuberosity*, the bump on your shin bone just below the kneecap.

You probably don't need to know this kind of nitty gritty, except that we sometimes refer to these terms in later chapters. Or if your orthopedist scans an x-ray and mutters something like "Ah ha, I see a problem with the tibial tuberosity!" you'll have some idea what he or she is talking about.

Growth Plates

Growth plates exist in many parts of the skeleton, and they come in two flavors: *Epiphyseal* plates add to the length of our

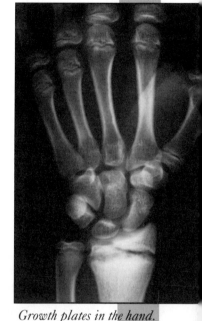

Growth plates in the hand. This x-ray shows the growth plates in the wrist and finger bones of an immature hand. The growth plates are the tiny dark transverse lines near the ends of all the bones. These lines disappear in adult x-rays. To compare this to an adult x-ray, see the chapter on the Shoulder, Elbow and Wrist. Note that this gymnast also has a stress fracture in the growth plate of the radius, the large forearm bone.

bones and make us grow taller, and *apophyseal* plates add to the thickness of our bones like the rings of a tree.

Because of the way growth plates change, they are the weakest part of a young person's bones, and susceptible to fracture. When growth comes to a halt in late adolescence, the growth plates turn into ordinary bone and become stronger.

Wolff's Law

This useful law states that bone responds to stress—or lack of it. In areas where bones are stressed, they become stronger; in areas where they aren't used, they become weaker. If you're stuck in a cast for a long time, the bone becomes weaker. But when you start working out again, it gets stronger.

As a fit gymnast, you not only have stronger muscles than someone who doesn't exercise, you also have stronger bones.

Fractures

A fracture can be anything from a microscopic crack in the bone to a total break. In an "open fracture," the kind they show in horror movies, the skin is broken, either by bone poking through it or by the blow that caused the fracture. This is also called a "compound" fracture. In a closed fracture, the skin is intact and the damage beneath is mercifully hidden from view.

Fractures can also be "displaced" or "non-displaced." A displaced fracture is the obvious kind because there are body parts bent at odd angles. Displaced fractures are the ones that must be "set" before being immobilized to heal.

Stress fractures of the tibia. The x-ray here shows two transverse lines representing stress fractures of the tibia in a 17-year-old gymnast.

16

Getting even nittier and grittier, here are further subcategories:

Greenstick fractures
These are breaks that go only part way through the bone—like cracking a green stick from a tree. These fractures happen only in children.

Comminuted fractures
Here the bone ends up in more than two pieces. Believe it or not, it's possible to pulverize the patella (knee cap) into several pieces, even though it's quite small to start with.

Stress fractures
Stress fractures start as tiny cracks and get worse if left untreated. This is not a little pain you can "work through."
Only humans, horses and greyhounds get stress fractures, and the common denominator is humans. It is humans who make horses and greyhounds run, and it is we humans who keep pushing ourselves long after our bodies cry *uncle.*
The good news is that in recovering from a stress fracture, the body normally responds by making the bone even stronger than it was. However, we do not recommend this as a way of generating strong bones.

Epiphyseal fractures
These fractures involve the growth plates at the ends of the long bones, which are weakened areas in children.

Apophyseal fractures
Here's a case where muscle is stronger than bone! Too much force on a tendon (and hence muscle) attached to an apophysis, and the apophysis can pop loose. Gymnasts are most likely to suffer problems from apophyses on the knee (Osgood-Schlatter disease—see the chapter on knees) or the heel (Sever Condition—see the chapter on the leg, ankle and foot).

By the way, it's an old wive's tale that a bone is only broken if you can't move it. Many broken bones still move fine—particularly stress fractures. Even a joint suffering a fairly severe fracture can still move.

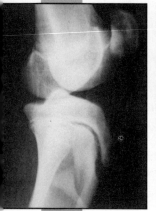 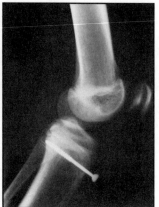

Avulsion of the tibial tubercle and surgical repair. The first x-ray of this Olympic gymnast's knee shows the growth plate pulled loose from the tibia. Jack used a screw to reattach the tubercle (as shown in the second x-ray), and the gymnast was back in training one week later.

JOINTS

Joints are the places bones come together. You knew that, right? But did you know that your skull has joints, too, where several bones fused shortly after you were born?

The joints we'll be talking about in this book are the ones that move. That movement depends on several components:

Articular Cartilage

Articular cartilage is the white, glistening cartilage that you see on the end of a chicken bone. It also covers the ends of your long bones, like the tibia and femur. Articular cartilage is very slippery, which enables joints to move without screeching and grating.

There is very little blood supply to the articular cartilage, so any damage heals slowly. If this cartilage gets worn away, bones can rub together and create irritation and inflammation. Eventually, you can get arthritis.

While the articular cartilage can absorb some shock, its main job is lubrication. Shock absorption falls to a different type

18

of cartilage: the *meniscus* in the knee and the spinal disc. We'll
have more to say about those in later chapters.

Synovial Fluid

Additional joint lubrication is provided by the "synovial
fluid" a thick liquid about the consistency of (following our
chicken analogy) egg white. The synovial fluid fills the joint
like motor oil in your car's crankcase. To keep the synovial fluid
from leaking out, the entire joint is encased in a sac called
(predictably) the "synovium."

Bursae

The bursae (if you're only talking about one of them,
it's a bursa) are sacs formed by two layers of synovial tissue and
filled with a dab of synovial fluid. It's the same idea as a jelly
doughnut. These little jobs appear at odd places in and around
joints to prevent friction between tendon and bone or skin
and bone.

Ligaments

We mentioned the synovium, the fluid-filled sac that
surrounds each joint. This sac is the inside layer of the joint
"capsule," the tough fibrous tissue that surrounds and supports
the joint. In some places the capsule is thin and flexible, which
allows the bones to move easily in certain directions; in other
places, the capsule is thick and tough, forming ligaments.
In simple terms, ligaments are the gristly bands that
hold bones together—tendons are the gristly ropes that attach
muscles to bones.
Some joints (the sacroiliac, for example) are surrounded
by thick ligaments and so have very little motion. At the

opposite extreme is the shoulder joint, which has few ligaments, a wide range of motion, and a correspondingly high risk of dislocation! (There are no free lunches.)

As we'll discuss in Body Types, people have ligaments of varying quality. Those with relatively loose, elastic ligaments will be the most flexible gymnasts.

Ligament Sprains

People talk all the time about spraining things, so let's get specific: If it's a ligament, you can *sprain* it; if it's a muscle, you can *strain* it; if it's a tendon, you can *tear* it.

Ligament sprains come in three grades. To get an idea, knit your fingers together tightly. This is the normal ligament with all the fibers snug against each other. Then:

- *Grade I (mild).* Stretched, but not broken. Loosen your fingers a bit. The fibers of the ligament are still intact, just looser.

- *Grade II (moderate).* Partially torn. Pull your hands apart some more, but keep your fingers touching. The fibers of the ligament are frazzled, and pain is more severe, but the ligament is mostly in one piece.

- *Grade III (severe).* Completely torn. Here your fingers do not touch. A ligament torn this badly cannot stabilize the joint, and it will have difficulty healing because the two torn ends may not be anywhere close to each other. Surgery is often (though not always) required. Oddly, a severe sprain may not have much pain associated with it as a moderate sprain, because the nerves are torn along with the ligament.

Dislocations

Any time a joint is so messed up that the bones don't come together the way they should, it's a dislocation. Dislocations typically mean torn ligaments, and they can also include fractured bones.

The joints most prone to dislocation are the shoulder, elbow, hip, ankle, and the small joints of the finger.

Chances are you will know right away if you dislocate a joint: First, it will look wrong. It will also be swollen, painful and difficult to move.

Bursitis

Anytime you see "itis" on the back of the name of something, you know that whatever it is, is inflamed. Bursitis is an inflammation of the bursa, caused by irritation and/or overuse. An inflamed bursa produces more fluid, swelling up and becoming still more painful. Gymnasts are somewhat prone to bursitis in their shoulders because they give their shoulders such heavy use.

If bursitis doesn't get better, or if it recurs, you should look harder for its cause. In the shoulder, it may be a bony impingement problem.

MUSCLES

We mentioned earlier that you have muscles you'll never be able to control. These are the involuntary muscles like the heart, the diaphragm and the little muscles that keep your intestines percolating.

Of course, you're interested in the voluntary, or skeletal muscles. In nearly every case, it takes several muscles, contracting or relaxing simultaneously, to accomplish even a simple motion.

21

All or nothing

Each muscle is made up of thousands of microscopic muscle fibers, and it is these little guys that contract. And for each one, contraction is an all-or-nothing deal. It either contracts to the max or not at all.

The way you achieve control is by varying the number of muscle fibers your nerves call into action. For the whole muscle, you have a great deal of control: You can contract it a little or a lot; you can lift a 5-lb weight or a 20-lb weight.

It may be that some athletes excel because their nervous systems can mobilize more muscle fibers to work together.

Tendons

Muscles attach to bones by means of tendons, ropy cords of fibrous tissue (gristle in your chicken dinner). Each muscle has an "origin" on a stationary bone and an "insertion" on the bone that it moves. Normally, the insertion tendon passes over the joint.

An example: The calf muscle that you see in the back of your leg originates on the posterior surfaces of the femur's condyles, just above and behind the knee joint. At the bottom of the calf muscle, the Achilles tendon passes behind the ankle and attaches to the heel bone. When you contract the calf muscle, you stand on your toes as the muscle shortens and the tendon pulls on the heel bone.

Aerobic and Anaerobic

We'll have more to say about this in the chapter on nutrition, but here's a muscle's-eye view. *Aerobic* muscle contraction uses an energy source known as ATP (adenosine triphosphate), plus oxygen. When ATP and oxygen get used up, an *anaerobic* process takes over: *glycolysis*. Glycolysis creates lactic acid (that nasty taste in your mouth when you get really winded), and it also creates an "oxygen debt." You can keep going quite a while with a mounting oxygen debt, but sooner or later that debt must be paid off (unlike the national debt). You have to rest so that the blood can resupply the muscle with oxygen and your body can get rid of all the lactic acid.

Muscle Strains

Sudden overload can tear the fibers of muscles and tendons, just as it can tear ligaments. This is called a muscle strain (not sprain). Like sprains, there are three grades of muscle strains, with the same descriptions.

Symptoms of strains include pain, muscle spasm and loss of strength. (For an explanation of how muscles go into spasm see the "Practical Guidelines for Flexibility Training" in the Training chapter.)

Tendinitis

Here's the classic overuse injury, made famous by "tennis elbow"—if not by "gymnast's wrist."

Although tendons are very strong, they get tired with repetitive exercise. Fatigue tends to occur where the tendon attaches to the bone, because the blood supply is especially poor here. A tired tendon is soon an inflamed tendon, and you are stuck with pain until it gets well.

Tendinitis can be acute or chronic. If you spend a day using a screwdriver, chances are you'll have a singing case of elbow tendinitis by nightfall. Tendinitis can also come on gradually like a stress fracture, which is particularly dangerous: You get used to the gradual increase of discomfort and don't get treatment, and in a few months, tendinitis has set up permanent housekeeping.

The moral with tendinitis is, don't ignore it or you won't be able to ignore it!

FIRST AID: RICE

Here is the most important first aid you need to know: RICE—Rest, Ice, Compression and Elevation. Just about any injury you may get in gymnastics will do better with a little RICE. And RICE will never hurt. So study this part of the book, and remember RICE the next time you get injured.

Rest

Stop using it! Do not run through the routine just one more time! If part of your body breaks, *give* it a break and rest it as soon as you realize an injury has happened.

If you continue to use an injured tissue you can make the injury much worse. You can also delay healing, cause more pain and stimulate bleeding. So the first thing to do is immobilize whatever part of you has been injured. Be careful how you do this—don't bend or twist anything!

To keep the injury immobilized, you may need to use crutches, splints, casts, braces or other aids. Until your trainer or doctor tells you it's OK to use something, stay off it.

Ice

The next step after getting *off* an injury is to get some ice *on* it. The sudden cold causes small blood vessels to contract, so less blood collects around the injury. The less blood, the less healing time. The ice will also help kill the pain. Here are some guidelines:

- For small injuries (finger, toe, foot or wrist), dunk it in a bucket of ice water.

- For larger injuries, use ice packs. A zip-lock plastic bag will do nicely. (Don't put ice directly on the skin, because the ice may be quite a bit colder than a mixture of ice and water, depending on the freezer it came from.) Apply the cold pack to the skin so that you numb the area completely. Don't use a towel between the ice and the skin, or the area won't get cold enough.

- Keep the ice in place for about 10-15 minutes. Then remove it and let the skin warm up. Repeat this two to three times per hour. Each time leave the ice in place until the area becomes numb.

- Repeat the cooling and warming cycles for a few hours—and follow the instructions for compression and elevation.

- If the injury swells up quickly, see your doctor as soon as possible, because the quick swelling means there are torn blood vessels and the injury is serious. Only blood can cause quick swelling—inflammation and other causes of swelling don't really show until a few days later.

- Keep using ice until the swelling begins to subside. That may happen in a day or in several days. In general, ice is the treatment of choice for the first 24 to 48 hours at least.

Compression

Compression is another way to decrease swelling by slowing bleeding and limiting the accumulation of blood and lymph. Without compression, fluid from nearby normal tissue seeps into the injury.

If possible, use an elasticized bandage. If you don't have one handy, use anything to wrap the injury. This is where you can be heroic and tear your T-shirt to help a friend. You can even wrap around the outside of the ice, so that the ice stays close enough to the skin to do its job.

Wrap firmly, but not too firmly. How do you know? If the limb below the wrap becomes numb or painful, or if muscles cramp, or if nails turn blue, you've overdone it. Unwrap until normal circulation returns, then re-wrap a bit more loosely.

Elevation

And here is yet another way to decrease the circulation of blood to the wound—elevate it above the level of the heart. This can really help decrease swelling and pain. You may have to be ingenious here, using pillows and whatever else you can find. You can help elevate the arm and shoulder by propping up the entire upper body, perhaps in a reclining chair or even a bed with two of its legs up on blocks.

COMMON DIAGNOSTIC TECHNIQUES

Yes, diagnostic techniques are not a basic part of your body, but they are basic to sports medicine. What other chapter could we put this in? We feel you should know something about the types of tests your doctor may order.

X-ray

The medical journals call x-rays "radiographic studies," maybe because everyone knows *x-ray* and it sounds so ordinary.

X-radiation travels through soft tissue but can't get past bone. When x-rays hit photographic film, they turn it black—just as film turns black if you pull it out of the canister in broad daylight. Wherever x-rays can't get to the film because a bone is in the way, the film remains clear. (It looks white when you hold it up in front of a light.)

X-rays are great at giving us a picture of a major bone break. But they don't show soft tissue problems, and they also don't show subtle bone problems. For example, most stress fractures won't show up on an x-ray film until at least 15 percent of the bone is missing from the hairline crack.

In addition, if you have a very complex bone structure, x-rays make it hard to tell exactly what is going on because they show everything at once.

Bone Scan

Bone scans can show stress fractures by showing where bone-building activity is taking place. To do a bone scan, the doctor will inject technetium-99, a radioactive substance that rushes around looking for *osteoblasts* to hide in. (Osteoblasts are the cells that build new bone.)

Of course, the technetium can't really hide because it's radioactive, so if you scan the body, the technetium shows up as bone-building "hot spots."

Doctors often use bone scans along with x-rays to tell if damage to a bone is new (lots of bone-building) or old (no hot spots).

Although this diagnostic technique uses radioactive material, it is not dangerous because the doses are very low and the radioactivity decays rapidly.

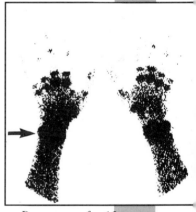

Bone scan of a 13-year-old gymnast's hands. This scan shows that the growth plates of the hands and wrists are still active. It also highlights the stress fracture of the left radius, shown in the previous x-ray of growth plates. This gymnast later competed in the Olympics.

27

Arthrogram

This is a way of looking at the joint capsule. It spotlights spaces.

To do an arthrogram, the doctor injects a radiopaque dye (this is a fluid that absorbs x-rays, as bone does) into the joint, often a shoulder joint. X-rays beaming through the joint show the bones and fluid on a TV monitor, and the doctor watches to see what happens to the fluid. If it leaks out of the joint, that can mean tears in the joint lining or in one of the joint's tendons or ligaments.

Linda has had a shoulder arthrogram and recommends watching the monitor along with your doctor. It keeps your mind off what is going on, and it's quite beautiful to see bones and joints in action from the inside out.

Arthroscopy

This new technology is changing the face of joint surgery. Instead of opening a joint with a four-inch incision, the surgeon makes a few tiny holes and works inside the joint with the minimum amount of disturbance.

The first hole, or portal, allows the surgeon to inject a clear fluid to expand the joint, provide a clear visual field, and give room to work. Once the joint is prepared, the surgeon inserts the arthroscope, an instrument that beams light into the joint (the miracle of fiber-optics) and relays an image back to a TV monitor. Looking at the screen, the surgeon inserts special miniaturized surgical instruments into other holes to carry out the actual repair.

Arthroscopy is extremely versatile, often allowing the surgeon to diagnosis and make the repair at the same time. Because arthroscopy uses only tiny incisions and leaves the joint mostly intact, recovery usually proceeds much faster than it does with conventional surgery.

Computerized Axial Tomography (CAT) Scan

A CAT scan (or CT scan) creates three dimensional x-ray images.

To have a CAT scan, you (or the body part in question) lie inside the large coil of a rotating x-ray tube. The rotating device emits x-rays, which are picked up by electronic sensors. The sensors feed data into a computer, which solves roughly a zillion complex mathematical equations and produces a single, three-dimensional x-ray image on a television monitor. The screen can be photographed, or the data can be saved on computer disk for future reference.

The advantage of a CAT scan is that it constructs a three-dimensional image, so it's a good way to visualize the interior of bones. The computer constructs the 3-D image from a whole series of sectional images, so it eliminates the problem of x-ray shadows. It's like taking a chunk of solid bacon, breaking it into slices to see exactly where the meat and fat are, and then reconstructing the slices into a single clean, precise 3-D image. If you just took one x-ray through the slab, you wouldn't be able to tell much.

Magnetic Resonance Imaging (MRI) Scan

Every atom in your body is like a child's top spinning around, wobbling slightly as it spins. And every type of atom has its own unique wobble. Magnetic Resonance Imaging (MRI) uses an immense uniform magnetic field to measure these different wobbles and show a picture of the body's tissues in fantastic clarity and detail.

The computer imaging technology behind MRI is quite similar to the CAT scan. Once again, you or your body part lie inside an impressive tubular deal. The difference is that instead of x-rays, the MRI uses a magnetic field. Leave your watch off!

The MRI can show soft tissues, like the discs between your spinal vertebrae or torn ligaments in your shoulder. The

MRI gives such a clear image, it is often used instead of an arthrogram to diagnose joint problems.

Isokinetic Measurements

We mentioned isokinetic exercise briefly in the chapter on training. But isokinetic ("constant motion") machines also have a diagnostic function.

These machines measure muscular strength and power. The machine is set to move at a maximum speed. The athlete works against the machine, and the machine records the power that the athlete develops. Isokinetic tests can reveal muscle weakness resulting from muscle or nerve damage, and they can also plot the progress that you make in rehabilitation after an injury.

SUMMARY

In this chapter, we've talked about the basic body building blocks that you rely on to carry you through your gymnastic career. The body is an incredible system, astoundingly resilient and capable of bouncing back from punishment that would destroy most human-made materials. In many ways, the body is stronger than steel: If you bend a piece of steel back and forth a few times, it snaps. But the human body repairs itself, gets stronger, and goes for more.

Nevertheless, there are limitations. Sometimes things break, or get fatigued or inflamed. Sometimes there is no substitute for rest and rehabilitation. We hope that if you know something about how your body works and when it needs help, you'll be a good friend to it. Your body is one of the best friends you'll ever have, and you want it to last a lifetime. Listen to it.

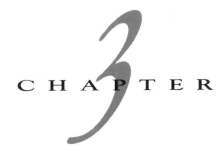

CHAPTER 3

Body Types

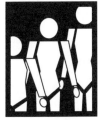

The body of a good athlete is like a well-tuned machine, perfectly matched to the job it faces. Since every sport uses the body a different way, it's not surprising to see different kinds of bodies excelling in different kinds of sports.

For example, marathon runners appear almost monotonously alike—tall and thin, greyhounds on a diet. They may look as if too many long runs have used them up, but the truth is that they have the perfect body for running marathons. Their long thin legs gobble up distance with great endurance, and there's no superfluous muscle or fat anywhere to add extra weight. Chances are most marathon runners looked a bit undernourished before they ever ran their first mile.

Now look at a different kind of runner. Check the line-up of rear ends before the gun goes off at a 100-yard dash. You'll note an impressive array of that largest muscle in the body, the gluteus maximus. Do sprinters have big buns because they eat too many french fries? No. It's because people with naturally hefty rear ends often make good sprinters. Those big muscles in back get them out of the blocks and up to speed in a hurry.

So what kind of body should you have if you want to be a gymnast?

First, let me say that there are no absolutes—talent and dedication make the best gymnast, not body type. And you can have a great time in gymnastics whether you're tall, short, fat or thin. Yet if you want to make it to the top ranks, certain body features will help.

Unlike sports such as marathon running, there is no one perfect type for gymnastics. When you're on the rings or the uneven bars, it helps to be built like a wrestler. When you're on the floor or the balance beam, it helps to be built like a ballet dancer. The best overall answer is somewhere in between.

So let's take a closer look at the whole subject. We'll start by finding out what kind of "morph" you are—one of those hereditary things. Then we'll talk about gears and levers, because that sentence about the body being a well-tuned machine is not idle chatter. If you understand a little about the physics of athletics, it's easier to understand why certain body types do better than others in certain sports.

Then we'll home in on muscles, bones and flexibility— and what you can and can't do to improve what you have.

Finally, we'll close with a few words about what to expect to happen to your body type as you go through puberty.

WHAT KIND OF MORPH ARE YOU?

Endo-, Ecto-, Meso-

In the animal kingdom, you see obvious relationships between size, shape and function. The elephant is huge, round, slow and powerful. The cheetah is lanky and fast. The gazelle is small, muscular, and nimble.

Humans fall into roughly the same three categories, with scientific names that make things sound more complicated than they really are:

■ *Endomorph*. This word comes from the Greek *endo*,
meaning within, and *morphe*, meaning form.
Endomorphic people tend to hang on to what they
eat. They have a natural tendency to gain body fat,
and they generally have a roundish look. Like the
elephant, endomorphs can excel where slow power is
required, like weightlifting. Of course, human
endomorphs are not elephants—the curvaceous ladies
that populate the Renaissance paintings of Rubens
show endomorphic loveliness at its most radiant.

■ *Ectomorph*. The word comes from the Greek *ektos*,
meaning outside. Ectomorphic people tend to turn
whatever they eat into energy. Like the cheetah, they
are thin and wiry. Ectomorphs can have trouble
gaining weight, and almost no amount of body-
building will give the true ectomorph the rippling
muscles that come naturally to the mesomorph. In
sports, ectomorphs win the endurance events.

■ *Mesomorph*. The word comes from the Greek *mesos*, or
middle. Roughly intermediate between the
endomorph and the ectomorph, the mesomorph is
compact and muscular, neither fat nor thin. The
mesomorph has a good ability to convert food to lean
body mass (muscles) and has a build that is square,
rather than round or long. Nimble and quick like the
gazelle, the mesomorph is a natural for gymnastics,
diving, pentathlon and other sports that require a
variety of skills.

Of course, almost no one is purely one body type or
another: We all have aspects from each category. One method of
describing physique is called the somatotype, which has three
numbers (for example, "5/3/2.5"). The first number indicates the
amount of endomorphy, the second the amount of mesomorphy,
and the third the amount of ectomorphy. Higher numbers

indicate a greater degree of that characteristic. The table here compares gymnasts to typical males and females.[1]

Somatotypes for gymnasts compared to non-athletes.

SOMATYPES FOR:	ENDOMORPHY	MESOMORPHY	ECTOMORPHY
Typical male (5/3/3)	5	3	3
Male gymnast (2/6/2)	2	6	2
Typical female (5/2.5/2.5)	5	2.5	2.5
Female gymnast (3/4.5/3)	3	4.5	3

Body Type and Body Fat

If you look at the winners in the top gymnastic events, you'll notice that they all look a lot alike: fairly small, lean and muscular. As the table indicates, most gymnasts are strongly mesomorphic, although many females have strong ectomorphic characteristics. Betty Okino typifies the ectomorphic type that excels in routines (like the balance beam) that stress gracefulness.

Gymnastic routines for boys (rings, parallel bars, pommel horse) put a special premium on muscularity.

The one type rare in high-level gymnastics is the person who is predominantly endomorphic. As we'll show in the chapter on nutrition, gymnasts have very little body fat: males generally have as little as four to six percent and females from eight to 15 percent. Normal males have 15 percent body fat and females 26 percent. It would

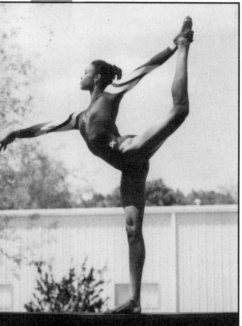

Photo courtesy of Leslie Spencer

An ectomorphic gymnast. Betty Okino is a good example.

be extremely difficult, if not impossible, for the staunch endomorph to reach the required low percentage of body fat.

(And of course, the reason the low percentage of body fat is so important is that you don't want to have to sling non-functional weight around.)

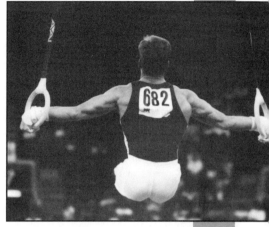

Muscularity Versus the Aesthetic Look

A mesomorphic gymnast. Mesomorphic muscularity really shows in this iron cross skill at the Goodwill Games.

Muscularity is obvious in a male gymnast as he carries out the iron cross on the rings, or speeds through the intricate maneuvers on the parallel bars or the pommel horse. Yet muscles can be equally important to females. It takes strong legs (and the buttocks of a sprinter!) to provide the explosive power required for the vault and floor acrobatics. And you can't tame the bars without powerful shoulders and arms.

Yet for girls in particular, too much muscularity can be something of a disadvantage. Muscles and flexibility don't naturally go together—the girl with plenty of muscles for the vault may not have the flexibility and gracefulness it takes for that back walkover on the balance beam.

There's also the aesthetic factor: Gymnastics, like dance, diving and figure skating, is such a subjectively judged activity that a certain amount of that "lean" look may be important. This is probably another reason gymnasts have so little body fat.

You may want to specialize in a part of gymnastics that favors your body type. If you're solidly mesomorphic and on the muscular side, go for the high-powered routines. If you tend to ectomorphic, specialize in events that require endurance and grace.

BODY MECHANICS: GEARS, LEVERS, TWITCHES, PROPRIOCEPTION

So far, we've talked about how certain bodies do certain things best. Now we want to say a bit about why that's so—the mechanics behind it.

Gears: Power Versus Speed

If you've ever ridden in a car, you're familiar with gears. The car starts in low gear with a lot of power to get all that metal moving—but low gear doesn't offer much in the way of ultimate high speed. If you stay in low gear, you'll be hard-pressed to top 30 mph.

As the car speeds up, your automatic transmission shifts into higher gears. At freeway speeds, in the highest gear, your car has plenty of speed, but very little reserve power. That's why the car drops into a lower gear when you jam the pedal to the metal to pass. It needs the extra power to accelerate quickly enough so you don't get converted to one of those depressing highway statistics.

The idea is that gears trade power for speed and vice versa. So you can use the same car to pull a heavy load slowly up a hill or to zoom through west Texas with insane disregard for the speed limit.

Human bodies, unfortunately, do not come with either automatic or manual transmissions. We are designed for a fairly narrow range of power and speed, and we can't swap gears. (Although we do have two "gears" of muscles, which we'll talk more about later.)

In general, people with short, thick muscles operate more in low gear: They are powerful and have the explosive energy to get moving fast from a standing start. But they are not so efficient at sustaining high output.

People with long thin muscles operate more in high gear: not too good from a standing start, but built for cruising and efficient expenditure of energy over long periods.

Mesomorphs tend to be low-gear people; ectomorphs, high-gear. The best gymnasts have some of each, but are predominantly low-gear mesomorphs.

Levers: Weight, Speed and Inertia

While the idea of gears helps understand how muscles work, the idea of levers helps explain the role of bones. Are you short–or tall? And how does that affect your performance in gymnastics? We're going to explain this in a way that will probably make university physics professors groan, but then they probably aren't going out for gymnastics anyway.

To get a quick idea of how levers work, go to the refrigerator and haul out a gallon of milk. Keep your arm at your side and lift it just by bending your elbow. Now keep your elbow straight and lift it by raising your whole arm—quite a bit more difficult!

When weight is out at the end of a long lever arm, it's harder to lift. The "effective weight" of the milk bottle has gone up because the "lever arm" is longer. Mathematically speaking, the idea is:

Effective weight = Actual weight x Length of lever arm

Since your entire arm from shoulder to wrist is about twice as long as your forearm, the effective weight of the milk is about twice as great if you lift it straight from the shoulder as it is if you bend your elbow.

Not only does it take more force to lift the milk with your arm straight, it's also a lot harder to do it *fast*. This relates to the problem of overcoming inertia. Inertia is the tendency of everything to stay just the way it is. It applies to just about everything, from getting your car up to speed after a stoplight, to slowing it down at the next light. It even applies to getting your body away from the TV set.

The formula for our milk-swinging example is:

$$\text{Inertia} = \text{Effective weight} \ \times \ (\text{Velocity})^2.$$

It takes energy to overcome inertia and get that gallon of milk really swinging from your shoulder. In fact, because velocity is squared in the formula, it takes *four* times as much energy to get the milk moving only *twice* as fast. And the milk is also harder to stop!

(If you are a gymnast trying this at home, make sure the lid is on tight—or that you have very good-natured parents!)

What do milk bottles have to do with gymnasts and body types? The longer your arms and legs are, the harder they are to move, the harder they are to move quickly, and the harder they are to stop moving.

The lever effect explains why the iron cross is so hard (especially if you have long arms), and inertia explains why pike maneuvers are tougher than tucks.

Gymnasts who make it to the top ranks are small people, with relatively short bones. The laws of physics simply make it easier for them to move their arms and legs quickly, precisely and with less energy.

Long bones may also predispose you to injuries. A foot at the end of a long leg will strike the mat with more force than a foot at the end of a short leg, even if the two gymnasts weigh the same and do exactly the same maneuver. And a long body whirling around the high bar has more inertia and exerts proportionately more force on the wrists, elbows and shoulders than a short body.

Muscle Twitches

We mentioned earlier that there are two "gears" within your muscles. Really, you have two types of muscle fibers, called "fast-twitch" and "slow-twitch." The fast-twitch fibers enable you to move quickly. They are what take you speeding down the runway.

Slow-twitch fibers handle slower tasks with great endurance. These fibers come into their own on the balance beam and during the slow parts of the floor routine.

Fortunately or unfortunately, to choose the correct amount of each muscle type to have, you have to choose your parents. Elite gymnasts will luck out with a high percentage of fast-twitch muscles, while the gold-medal marathoner will star in the slow-twitch category.

Regardless of your own particular brand of twitchiness, be sure to work both of these muscle types by including both fast and slow exercises in every workout.

Proprioception: Do You Know Where You Are?

Here's a trick to try: Stand with your eyes closed and your arms out to the side, index finger pointed. Now bring your hands together and see if you can touch your two index fingers together, without opening your eyes. If you can, you have good "proprioception," which means that you know where your body is, even if you're not looking at it. This is a real handy talent for aspiring gymnasts, because you certainly can't keep looking at every part of your body during a routine! Proprioception also means you have good balance.

Of course, your proprioception will improve with training, too, so if you're not a natural, don't despair.

Another test of proprioception is to stand on one leg with your eyes closed and see how long you can balance without putting the other foot down. As you progress in gymnastics, this should become easier and easier.

COLLAGEN: THE SECRET OF FLEXIBILITY

While you are choosing your parents for muscles that twitch the way you want, go ahead and pick out parents with extremely elastic collagen. Because that's the secret of flexibility, one "must have" for gymnastics.

What is Collagen?

Perhaps you've heard of collagen—it's right there in the cosmetic ads, along with mink oil, bee pollen, crushed cucumber and aloe vera juice. As far as we know, collagen doesn't do much smeared on the outside of the skin, but inside the body, where it occurs naturally, it is a critical ingredient in muscles, tendons and ligaments. Collagen is a key factor in holding your skeleton together.

If you have naturally elastic collagen, your muscles will stretch easily. The ligaments holding your bones together (the joint capsule) will also stretch easily, so you can get your body into positions that cause normal people to wince and turn pale.

By the way, "double-jointed" people really don't have odd joints—they just have extra stretchy collagen. If you love gymnastics and you're double-jointed, you're extra-lucky, so pat yourself on the back. You're one of the few people who can do that without dislocating anything!

Determining Your Flexibility

Here's a quick test to assess the elasticity of your collagen: Use one hand to bend the thumb of the other hand toward your wrist. Bend it inward, toward the soft side of the arm—not the hairy side where your watch is.

If you want to do well in gymnastics, your thumb should touch your arm fairly easily. The easier the better. If you can't even get close, well, you may want to consider another sport.

Building and Maintaining Flexibility

If you're starting gymnastics at a young age, under ten, you should be quite flexible. Most kids are. Make sure your workouts include static stretches (see the chapter on exercises), to help maintain your flexibility as you grow older. Concentrate especially on the back, hip, hamstrings and shoulders, which all need to be very flexible in gymnasts.

Unfortunately, flexibility depends heavily on heredity, and if you're not naturally flexible, especially as a youngster, you probably never will be. It's just one of those things.

THE CHANGING BODY

Wouldn't it be great if you could start gymnastics with one body type, size and shape and never worry about it changing! As it is, it seems that as soon as you perfect a routine, something *grows* and throws everything off. It's all part of the challenge.

Growth Plates

We grow as our bones grow longer and bigger around. Most of this growth happens at certain places in the bones called *growth plates*. For more information on growth plates, see the section in Body Basics.

If your growth plates are open, you're still growing and will get taller. Once you reach your final height, the plates close, and that's it.

If you're desperate to know how much growth you have coming, your doctor can give you an estimate using x-rays to evaluate your growth plates. Basketball players are always delighted when their plates are still open; teenage gymnasts, when their plates close up.

Puberty

Here are the mega-changes, springing up in no apparent order, in no orderly time frame. It's hard to know what to expect and exactly when to expect it.

Linda's son ran with a crowd of teenagers all about the same size, except for one boy who remained steadfastly short, skinny and beardless while everyone else was bulking up and growing hair. The parents of this boy begged him to eat. At about the age of 18, years after the rest of the gang had mostly finished growing, everything kicked in for this kid. Today, he looks down on all of them.

So if you don't fit your friends' pattern, keep the faith. It will all work out in the end. Don't give up on a sport just because you don't have the perfect body type today. Maybe next month you will.

Having said that everyone is different, let me now throw in some averages.

- Boys generally start maturing between the ages of 13 and 16. During puberty the percentage of body fat goes down, shoulders widen and muscles develop— all to the advantage of the aspiring gymnast.

- Girls usually start puberty between 11 and 13. As girls progress through this period, their percentage of body fat tends to increase and their pelvis widens, neither of which makes gymnastics any easier. The widening pelvis changes the angle from hip to knee to toe; this change in biomechanics can mean that you'll have to rework some routines to compensate. In some cases, the increased angle can create knee problems. (See the chapter on The Knee and Thigh.)

SUMMARY

This chapter has explained the different body types and, we hope, some of the reasons why some body types are better in certain sports.

Regardless of all the body types, the best type of body for you is the one you have. Especially since you can't change it. Why feel bad about something that can't be changed? Enjoy your body, love it, take care of it. And have fun, whatever sports you get involved in and however far you progress!

---

[1] Fox, E.L.: Sports Physiology. Philadelphia, W.B. Saunders, 1979.

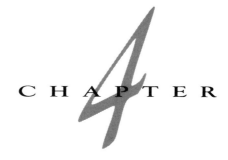

Nutrition

Relax, this is not a lecture on the four food groups.
What it is, is some information about nutrition that's
especially pertinent for gymnasts. Why should you be
different from other athletes? Several reasons:

■ You're young. That means that you're still growing, so
besides the nutrition your body needs for gymnastics, you also
need proper nutrition to grow. You have a much greater need
for calories than a mature athlete expending the same amount
of energy.

■ You're in a sport that requires more muscles than endurance.
That means you want muscles without fat. Fat means more
weight to throw around, and it's already hard enough throwing
around what you have.

■ You're in a sport where appearance can count. Dieting to look
wispy, of course, isn't the obvious path to the body of steel.
Which is what you need to carry off the moves.

■ Your training is unusual, to say the least. Your workouts
alternate short periods of extreme exertion (anaerobic activity)
with rest periods and lower exercise levels. It's not the typical
kind of sustained aerobic workout that most athletes use.

In this chapter, we'll talk about the role of diet in gymnastics, the various nutrients (and how much of each you need), vitamin supplements, and fluid replacement during exercise.

Then we'll focus on diet and weight control and some of the unpleasant things that can happen if you get compulsive about losing weight. There's a big difference between controlling weight and controlling body fat. We'll have a lot to say about listening to your body, which is a good thing.

THE ROLE OF DIET IN GYMNASTICS

First, forget fads. There is no magic diet that will make you a star. Diets don't create strong, agile bodies; strength and agility come only through training. But your diet gives your body the raw material it needs to construct the strong, agile body you want. So your diet must be *complete*.

Look at it this way: If you were running an automobile assembly line, you'd have a hard time turning out cars if you had no wheels or windshields, never mind how flashy the leather interior or how radical the instrumentation. Likewise, a good diet has to include all the essential nutrients. Grapefruit alone won't do it.

How Much of What?

The body needs six kinds of nutrients: carbohydrates, proteins, fats, vitamins, minerals and water. (Contrary to popular belief, chocolate is not an essential nutrient.) Carbohydrates, proteins and fats give you energy, while vitamins, minerals and water keep the body machinery humming to deliver that energy. In scientific terms, they support the enzymes and hormones that carry out the chemical reactions that make everything happen.

Carbohydrates, proteins and fats are the "crude oil" from which your body's gasolines—glucose and fatty acids—are refined. Glucose is a special form of sugar that comes from carbohydrates and proteins. Fatty acids come from proteins and fat.

In simple terms, you should get about 60 percent of your calories from carbohydrates, 15 percent to 20 percent from proteins, and the rest from fat (20 to 25 percent). We'll say more later about some practical ways to do this.

Exercise and fuel

There are two forms of exercise, aerobic and anaerobic. They use the body's fuels in vastly different ways:

Aerobic exercise

Aerobic means that the muscles use oxygen slowly enough to allow the blood to continually replenish the supply. You breathe hard, but you aren't gasping. (If you can't talk, you're not aerobic.) Aerobic exercise burns fat, and some sugar.

Pure sugar does two things: (1) It gives an immediate, but short, energy boost; and (2) it increases your insulin level. (Insulin is the enzyme that your body uses to burn sugar for energy.) The extra insulin burns up all the sugar and then looks around for more, making you feel hungrier than ever. Even worse, the increased insulin blocks the enzymes that make fat available as fuel, so the fat campfire starts to go out! Depressing, isn't it?

Anaerobic exercise

Anaerobic means that your muscles have essentially used up all the free oxygen, and the blood can't deliver enough in time. Without oxygen, the muscles can't burn fat; they must find some other fuel. The first thing the muscles go after is glycogen, a stored form of sugar. Some glycogen sits in the muscles themselves, where it makes a handy energy supplement.

Glycogen also resides in your liver; in order for this glycogen to get to the muscles, the blood must take it there. In anaerobic exercise, the muscle is already working so hard that the blood supply isn't adequate. This means that glycogen is not a long-term solution for anaerobic energy needs. What the muscle burns is—muscle. Not great, if you're trying to build more!

49

The point is, yes, your gymnastics routines are often anaerobic, and that can't be helped. But it's hard on the body and it doesn't burn fat or build muscle.

Carbohydrates

Carbohydrates include sugars, starches and fibers, in foods like rice, cereals, whole-grain bread, pasta, vegetables and fruits. One gram of carbohydrate yields four calories. (Remember this. You'll need it later.)

The body converts sugars and starches to glucose for energy or glycogen for energy storage.

Fiber keeps your intestines functioning smoothly and helps prevent constipation, heart disease, cancer of the colon and diabetes. Do not look down on that bran muffin.

About 60 to 65 percent of the calories in your diet should be carbohydrates. Contrary to popular opinion, potatoes will not make you fat. Only the butter, sour cream and cheese that make them taste so good do that.

Proteins

Proteins are long chains of amino acids, chemicals that contain nitrogen. Nature has 22 amino acids to work with, and from this, manufactures a seemingly infinite number of special purpose proteins. Some become enzymes, some hormones, some are structural components of the cells of your body. And of course, some become muscles. When protein is used for energy, one gram yields four calories, the same as carbohydrates.

The body, resourceful as ever, can use proteins for energy by converting them to fatty acids or glucose.

Proteins come to us in meat, fish, eggs, beans, nuts and dairy products. Vegetables have proteins too, although they generally do not have all 22 flavors. That's why vegetarian diets can lack important nutrients.

Only ten to 15 percent of the total calories you eat should come from protein. The body can't store it, and anything more than this just goes into energy storage or *fat*.

50

Although athletes may need a little more protein than non-athletes, the typical American diet exceeds the amount of protein that gymnasts require. Furthermore, high protein diets can be hard on the kidneys. Balance is important: If your diet is not balanced, or if your caloric intake is too low, your body will use protein for energy rather than building muscle. This is why carbohydrates are so important.

Fats

Fats include many categories. One you've heard about is cholesterol, one of the sterols. The category we're concerned with here is triglycerides, the major storage form of fats, which consists of glycerol and three fatty acids. Now here's the thing about fat: One gram of fat yields *nine* calories. This is the body's favorite way of storing energy, because it is so *efficient*. To lose one pound of fat, you have to burn *more than twice as many calories* as you do to lose one pound of glycogen or protein.

Fats appear mostly in foods we love: ice cream and chocolate, plus meats, eggs, whole milk, cheese, fried foods, butter, margarine, salad dressing, oils, and mayonnaise, to name a few. Brussels sprouts have no fat.

High fat intakes are associated with heart disease, cancer of the colon, breast cancer, and overall fatness. As a gymnast, you should try to keep the fat content of your diet between 20 and 25 percent of your total calories. And remember, when you figure calories, a gram of fat gives you more than twice the calories of a gram of carbohydrate or protein. Not fair, is it?

Vitamins

The Food and Nutrition Board of the National Research Council states that a proper mix of food should provide adequate amounts of vitamins and minerals. However, it's probably a safe thing to take a multiple vitamin supplement every day.

Now some people think if a little is good, a lot will be better, so they take megavitamin doses. We don't believe this is helpful; in some cases it simply creates very expensive urine, and in other cases, it can be dangerous.

Let me explain: Vitamins are either soluble in water or in fat...

Water-soluble vitamins

The key water-soluble vitamins are B complex and C. Too much niacin (a B-complex vitamin) can cause fatigue, tingling, flushed skin and liver damage. However, megadoses of the other water soluble vitamins do not appear to be toxic. The body simply gets rid of the overload by dumping excess vitamins into the urine. All that money, down the drain.

Fat-soluble vitamins

The fat-soluble vitamins are another story. These are vitamins A, D, E and K, and they remain in your body, especially in your liver, until your body uses them. If you eat more than you can use, they accumulate. And if too much accumulates, you get toxic symptoms. Too much vitamin A, and you can die.

So it is especially important not to overdose on fat-soluble vitamins.

Minerals

Minerals fall into two categories: major and trace.

Major minerals include calcium, iron, magnesium, potassium and sodium. You need relatively large amounts of these minerals—more than 100 mg a day.

Trace minerals include chlorine, chromium, copper, fluorine, iodine, manganese, molybdenum, phosphorus, selenium, sulfur and zinc.

With a few exceptions, mineral supplements aren't generally necessary. The exceptions can include calcium, iron, zinc and potassium.

If you eat enough dairy products (at least three to four glasses of milk a day), you should get enough calcium. If you hate milk, consider low-fat yogurt or cottage cheese. Otherwise take a calcium supplement.

Menstruating women should eat plenty of iron-containing foods (for example, spinach, flank steak, figs, turkey, baked beans, pork loin) or take an iron supplement, since iron is the absolutely critical part of the hemoglobin in the blood. Hemoglobin carries oxygen; without enough oxygen circulating, you won't have the energy you need.

Potassium is a salt like sodium that your body loses when you sweat. Foods rich in potassium include bananas, orange juice and cereals. You could also consider a small daily supplement of potassium. We'll have more to say about potassium when we talk about water and fluid loss.

Water

The human body is 65 percent water, and it just doesn't work well with less. You must replace fluid loss during exercise. In normal activities, most people don't suffer from a water deficiency.

Remember how we have been talking about "burning" sugar and fat for energy? When you burn fuel, you generate heat, just like a fire that burns wood. If your body doesn't get rid of that heat, you can cook to death. That's what happens when people have heat stroke. Water keeps you from getting too hot by evaporating from your skin. If you don't replace that water, you lose your ability to stay cool!

Weigh yourself before and after exercise and see how much water you lose. Then drink two cups for every pound lost.

How sweat works
The main way your body gets rid of heat is to sweat. Why does this work? Because it takes a lot of heat to turn water from a liquid to a vapor. (Just think of how long you heat a pot of water before it boils.) Your body cools itself through the vaporization of sweat. Every drop of sweat that evaporates carries heat with it.

A normal person in an hour-long aerobic dance class will burn about 300 calories, and the heat will be carried off by about a pint (two cups) of sweat. People who exercise harder (like gymnasts) burn more calories and generate more sweat.

Water replacement

You can't make sweat unless you have the water to do it. So you must continually replace water during your workouts! As little as two percent dehydration will impair your body's ability to regulate temperature. And at only three percent dehydration, your muscles lose endurance.[2]

One thing that complicates water replacement is that when you're working hard, most of your blood is in your muscles, not your digestive system. If you drink a lot of water all at one time, your body will have a hard time soaking it up. So load up on water before you start your workout, and then take a few sips every few minutes as you go along. Don't worry about having to go to the bathroom too often—remember, this water is for sweat, not urine.

Be sure to drink cool water. That's another way to help keep your body from overheating.

Special "exercise" fluids

But what about Gatorade® and other drinks that replace "lost electrolytes?" Recent literature is divided on the use of these supplemental drinks. We don't think you need them unless you have upped your workout and your sweat tastes particularly salty. While your body acclimates to the new routine, you may need a little extra salt—both sodium *and* potassium—and supplemental drinks can provide it. Supplements with sugar shouldn't be necessary unless you exercise more than one hour at a stretch.

For more information on sports nutrition information, write to the Gatorade Sports Science Institute, P.O. Box 049005, Chicago, Illinois 60604-9005, telephone 312-222-7704.

DIET AND WEIGHT CONTROL

As a gymnast, you may worry about your weight for two reasons: First, you want to look good. Second, an increase in weight changes your momentum and throws off your timing. So chances are, you're trying not to gain weight, and you may even be trying to lose it.

There are two ways to control your weight: diet and exercise. To be effective, diet and exercise must work together—too much emphasis on one or the other, and you can really run amuck.

In this section, we'll start by reviewing some of the unpleasant side effects of too much dieting. Then we'll look at a new way of looking at weight control by looking at *fat control*. Then we'll get specific about how you can improve your diet.

Watch Out For That Diet!

Did you know that too much dieting can stunt your growth? Do you want to grow up to be a midget? Constant dieting can lead to deficiencies in vitamins and minerals; not only does this lead to retarded growth, it also lowers your athletic performance and endurance.

Excessive dieting is especially hard on calcium uptake, and calcium is absolutely required for strong bones. Recent research[3] shows that the bone density of anorexic women is the same as that of 60-year-old women. If you get too carried away with dieting, you could be making your bones old and frail long before their time.

Iron levels also suffer from excessive dieting. Without iron, your blood can't get oxygen to your muscles, so you feel weak and lousy, you perform poorly, and you tend to injure yourself.

Even worse, people who become obsessed with dieting can easily become anorexic or bulimic.

Anorexia nervosa
This is a condition that is both psychological and physical. Anorexics develop such a phobia against food, that

they are often unable to eat, even when their bodies are starving for food. Left untreated, anorexics can die from the disease.

The adolescent gymnast (usually female) can become anorexic when she gets so obsessed with a thin body image that no amount of thinness seems to be enough. When she looks at herself in the mirror, it's as though she's looking in one of those fun-house mirrors that make everyone look fat. No matter how emaciated she is, she finds some lump of "fat" that needs to come off.

You may have anorexia if you:

- Think about food or dieting constantly or obsessively.

- Are continually depressed and feel fat, even when your weight is low or decreasing.

- Lose weight when there is no medical reason.

- Have no desire to keep your weight up to the recommendations of your trainers.

- Have irregular periods or no periods at all.

If you even suspect you might have anorexia after reading this, run—don't walk—to a physician or dietitian for professional help. You may also need extensive psychological counseling. This is not a condition to be ignored, and it's best to catch it in the early stages!

Bulimia

Like the anorexic, the bulimic is obsessed by food, dieting and weight control, but in a somewhat different way. This person binges on food—often consuming astounding quantities—and then vomits it back to avoid gaining the weight. Vomiting can even become an addictive behavior. Sometimes bulimics use laxatives excessively to prevent the intestine from doing the normal job.

While this behavior may combine to achieve a "normal" weight, it is *extremely* damaging to the body. You need immediate professional help to adopt healthy eating patterns and possibly save your life.

Fat Control vs. Weight Control

Weight is easy to measure, but it's not a very good way to determine body fitness. Weight includes bone, muscle, water, fat and other tissues. But obviously a person who has most of the weight in muscle is much better off than the one who has most of the weight in fat, even if they weigh the same!

By the way, muscle weighs more than fat. So you can be building muscle and trimming down the size of your body and be *gaining weight at the same time!* Obsessing about your weight can get you depressed when you should be elated.

Measuring body fat

The best way of keeping tabs on your body is to monitor your percentage of body fat. Unfortunately, there is no such thing as a body fat monitor you can step on every morning in the bathroom.

Body fat can be measured three ways: Immersion in water, skinfold measurement by calipers, and electrical impedance. The immersion method is the most accurate, but quite complex and expensive. Calipers measure the thickness of skinfolds in certain areas of the arms and abdomen. The thickness depends on the amount of fat under the skin, which is a good indication of total body fat. The electrical impedance method measures the flow of a tiny current of electricity through the body and uses a computer to calculate body fat.

If you are a serious gymnast, your trainer or coach should have some method for keeping tabs on your percentage of body fat. That way, as you gain weight (as growing individuals are bound to do) you can relax because you'll be able to tell that it's going into new muscles, not flab.

How much is too much?

The "standard" amount of body fat for a "normal" adult female is 26 percent; for a male, 15 percent. Athletes have less, and gymnasts have the least of all: about five percent for males and nine to 17 percent for females.[4] If you are striving for these low levels of body fat, you should be professionally monitored to make sure you do not fall too low.

A Nutrition Plan That Works

A nutrition plan will only work if you personalize it to your needs and your likes and dislikes. Some recommended diet may be wonderful, but if broccoli is a big feature and you can't stand broccoli, forget it.

The best plan is to analyze what you eat now and take a close look at what you want to attain. Then make small gradual changes to migrate to a healthy eating style that you can maintain for your whole life. The main thing is to avoid another dreadful diet. Instead, figure out how to feed yourself healthfully.

By the way, it's a myth that the less you eat, the faster you'll lose weight. Starving yourself only makes you hungrier, and sooner or later you'll compensate by going on a binge. Then you'll feel guilty and starve yourself even worse. . .and so on.

How does your present diet measure up?
Take an honest look at your current food choices. For four days, keep track of what and how much you eat—everything that goes in your mouth. Include weekend days as well as week days. Write it all down for each meal: what you ate and how much. Don't forget those between-meal snacks! Then summarize the results:

- Ounces of meat per day: (three ounces is equivalent to one regular hamburger, one chicken breast, one chicken leg (thigh and drumstick), one pork chop or three slices of pre-sliced lunch meat.)

- Servings of breads and cereals per day, preferably whole-grain: (One serving is one slice of bread, one ounce of cereal, or one-half cup cooked cereal, pasta, rice or grits.)

- Fruit: (One serving is a whole piece of fruit, one-half cup juice, one-half grapefruit, one-quarter melon, one-half cup cooked or canned fruit, one-quarter cup dried fruit.)

- Vegetables: (One serving is one-half cup cooked or chopped raw vegetable or one cup leafy raw vegetable.)

- Cheese per day or week: (One serving is one ounce. Note low-fat or regular.)

- Milk per day: (One serving is one cup. Note skim, low-fat, whole.)

- Egg yolks per week:

- Lunchmeat, hot dogs, corned beef, sausage, bacon, other highly processed meats per week:

- Baked goods and ice cream (cake, cookies, coffee cake, donuts, etc.):

- Servings of snack foods per day or week (chips, fries, party crackers):

- Spreads used per day: (One serving is one pat of butter or one tablespoon of salad dressing.)

Guidelines for healthy eating

Now that you've kept track for four days, compare the results to these guidelines for a healthy diet. Each day you should have:

- Two to three servings of meat, for a daily total of about six ounces. This also includes eggs, although you should limit your eggs to four per week. Dried peas and beans can be substituted for meat.

- Six to 11 servings of bread, cereals, rice or pasta, preferably whole-grain products.

- Two to four servings of fruit.

- Three to five servings of vegetables.

■ Three to four servings of dairy products, which should be low-fat.

■ Three or fewer margarine or other "spread" servings.

■ Minimal snacks and sweets!

A healthy diet will have little obvious fat in it. You won't see mounds of chips and crackers or pounds of cheese. (Did you know that cheese is about 75 percent fat?) You won't see gallons of ice cream either, or french fries or fast food. Even though you don't set out to eat fat, you can be sure that your diet will still have enough to meet your nutritional needs.

This may all sound very difficult to achieve, but the trick is to take it one step at a time. Remember that you aren't trying to achieve perfection overnight—that isn't possible. Instead, you are trying to establish healthy eating habits that will stand by you for a lifetime.

DEVELOPING A SUCCESS STRATEGY

Once you have a baseline (the analysis of your current eating habits) and a goal in mind, you can build a sensible eating plan. Remember, no plan is cast in concrete. Chances are you will want to modify your diet as you go along, based on how well it works for you.

Plan your calories so that at least 60 percent come from carbohydrates (that's complex carbohydrates like vegetables, cereal and pasta, not sugar); ten to 15 percent from protein; and no more than 25 percent from fat.

Don't try to eliminate all the fun foods. Instead of forbidding yourself that piece of Chocolate Decadence Double Fudge Cake, have a small piece. Think about *how much* you eat, not just *what* you eat.

Here are some tips to get you started.

Listen to Your Body

The most important thing about eating sensibly is staying in touch with your body while you eat. Some people get so obsessed with counting calories, they lose the ability to tell when they're hungry or full. Overweight people typically continue to eat when they are not hungry, especially at night.

The next time you feel like you've just *got* to put something in your mouth, ask yourself if you're really hungry. Or are you bored or angry or lonely. Eating cannot help any of these other problems.

Eat slowly to give your body a chance to absorb the food—that's the only way it can tell you when it's had enough! *Stop eating when you feel comfortable, NOT when you feel full.*

Remind yourself that food is close by somewhere, and if starvation feels imminent, you can always eat again.

Use your diet as a tool. Practice it. Experiment. How much of what makes you feel comfortable? What makes you hungry? How long does a certain type of food "stick with you"?

Forget that stuff about "cleaning your plate." Mothers have been saying that for centuries (along with the part about starving children). That's a terrible way to learn about how to nourish your body!

Listen to your cravings, too. When you crave an orange, go eat one! Our bodies are very clever in telling us what they need, if we're clever enough to listen.

Watch Those Fats!

First determine your fat allowance. Experts recommend that the general population get no more than 30 percent of their calories from fat. We recommend that gymnasts keep this to 20 to 25 percent Currently, the average person in the U.S. gets about 37 to 40 percent of their calories from fat!

Most processed food packages show the number of grams of fat in the food. But how do you figure out the total grams of fat that are right for you?

Calculating your fat allowance

First, figure out how many calories you burn each day. The figure is 2,000 calories a day for a moderately active woman and 2,500 to 3,000 calories a day for a moderately active man. The number of calories you burn depends on your age, sex and how much you exercise. One three-day nutritional survey of female gymnasts showed that the caloric consumption per day ranged from 1,283 to 2,478 with a mean of 1,744.[5] These girls averaged about 15 years old and were club level A gymnasts. Get your trainer or coach to help you with this, or see the section about finding professional help.

Second, do a bit of math:

■ Multiply the percent of calories from fat times the total number of calories. For example, if you want to keep your fat intake at 20 percent of total calories and your total calories per day is 2,000, the formula is: .2 x 2000 = 400 calories from fat.

■ Divide the number of fat calories by nine. (Remember that one gram of fat gives you nine calories?)

400 calories ÷ nine calories per gram = 44.4 grams of fat.

Third, watch the labels and keep your fat consumption under 45 grams per day. Consider buying a fat gram counter to help you learn where hidden fats lurk. You can often find these at the grocery checkout counter. The T-Factor fat gram counter is one we can recommend.

Fat content of typical foods[6]

Listing the fat content of most foods would take a book in itself, but here are some samples. As you can see, fat is almost everywhere!

■ One tablespoon of salad dressing (or one big pat of butter) contains 13.three grams of fat (120 calories).

■ A large egg has five to six grams of fat per yolk.

- Two tablespoons of cream cheese (about one ounce) has ten grams of fat and only two grams of protein.

- A quarter-pounder with cheese has about 31 grams of fat. A small quarter-pound hamburger has about 11 grams.

- One raised donut has about ten grams.

- One-half cup of gourmet ice cream has 20 grams of fat! (This is really depressing.)

- Two slices of bologna has about 15 grams.

- One medium croissant has about ten grams.

- Three chocolate chip cookies have about ten grams.

- One ounce of potato chips has about ten grams.

Ten ways to cut fat[7]

Some fairly simple measures can make a significant difference in the fat that gets into you. Here are ten of them:

- Drink skim milk.

- Eat whole-grain breads, which taste good without butter.

- Use jam and jelly instead of butter on toast and rolls.

- Eat more pasta, rice and vegetables.

- Eat lean meat, fish and poultry. Remove skin from chicken!

- Use a vegetable as an entree instead of meat.

- Use low-fat or fat-free salad dressings. The new ones taste fine.

■ Snack on fruit or carrot sticks, unbuttered popcorn and pretzels instead of fried chips, crackers and cookies.

■ For dessert, choose fruit, angel food or sponge cake. Use fruit purees as icing.

■ Substitute low-fat or frozen yogurt for ice cream. Try frozen juice bars.

Eat like a "10"

Start with small changes. Identify a fatty food you can do without fairly easily, and do without it. Next week, pick out another. And so on. Don't even try to do it all at once—that's like trying a routine on the high bar before you've even mastered the walkover. Every goal worth achieving takes time.

Keep track of your progress. Record the changes you make and compare them to your ultimate goal. Give yourself a pat on the back (not a pat of butter) for your small successes. Remember, this is a program of progress, not perfection. This is not some diet that will be over with next Wednesday—this is a new way of life. So keep it pleasant.

Eating for the Big Event: To Load or Not To Load?

You may have heard of carbohydrate loading. The idea behind it is to force the body to store extra glycogen in the muscles, so the glycogen can supply energy in endurance events. People have developed elaborate schemes to turn carbohydrates into muscular glycogen. Most of these schemes include exercising to exhaustion (or fasting) to deplete glycogen stores, then tanking up on spaghetti and other carbohydrates.

Gymnasts simply shouldn't use these extreme forms of carbohydrate loading. For one thing, gymnastics is not an endurance event. Unlike the marathon runner, you are not going full blast for a couple of hours.

64

Second, fasting or exhaustion exercise can be very hard on the body. It may cause more damage than any possible benefit you can get from loading up afterwards.

The food you eat immediately before an event does not generally improve performance—that comes from your dietary habits for the past several months! The meals right before the Big Event should not contain high-protein or high-fat foods. They take longer to digest, and they increase the stress on the kidneys. The best meal is one rich in carbohydrates.

Here are some guidelines:

- Eat solid food three to four hours before the event, or drink a liquid meal two to three hours before. The liquid meal should be low-fat, low-protein and with some vitamins and minerals.

- Avoid anything that causes gas! You don't need jet propulsion.

- Don't eat sweets or sugared drinks within one hour of the meet. The insulin they stimulate will eat up your glycogen!

- Be sure to drink enough to stay hydrated.

Still Puzzled? How to Get Professional Advice

A registered dietitian is expert who can separate facts from fads when it comes to food and nutrition. You'll find them at work in many areas of our lives—with food companies, in sports medicine centers, hospitals, health clubs, research laboratories, daycare facilities and senior citizens' centers.

To locate a registered dietitian, ask your doctor or call the local hospital. You can also write to the National Center for Nutrition and Dietetics, 216 West Jackson Boulevard, Suite 800, Chicago, Il 60606-6995.

For more information, see the chapter on the Medical Team.

SUMMARY

This chapter contains so much material, it may be hard to assimilate all at once. Maybe that's just as well. One of the key points here is to approach diet rationally, one step at a time. Make small changes and listen to your body. Stay away from fads and give yourself credit for everything you do that's right, regardless of how small or insignificant it may appear to be. If you even suspect that you are getting obsessive about food or your weight or your body, talk to your coaches right away!

[2] McArdle WD, Katch FI, Katch VL. Exercise physiology. Philadelphia: Lea & Febiger, 1986; 451-453.

[3] Crosby L, Kaplan F, Pertshuk MJ, Mullen JL. The effect of anorexia nervosa on bone morphometry in young women. Clin Orthop & Rel Res, 1985; 201:271-277.

[4] Wilmore JH, "Body Composition and Athletic Performance, Nutrition and Athletic Performance," (Palo Alto, Calif.: Bull Publishing Co., 1981.

[5] Calabrese LH, "Nutritional and Medical Aspects of Gymnastics," Clinics in Sports Medicine, 4:1, Jan 1985.

[6] Hackman, EM, "Eating for your heart's content," Changing Times Magazine Supplement.

[7] Tribole E, "Eat Right America," Supplement to the Journal of the American Dietetic Association.

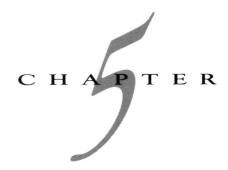
Training

Training—the very heart of gymnastics. So let's make it a real love affair!

Look at it this way: 99 percent of the time you won't be performing in front of the cheering throngs or even in front of your adoring parents. Instead, you'll be training to do it. So besides being effective, your training program should be *enjoyable*. One great reason to get involved in a sport is that you can't live without the fun of practice.

In this chapter, we'll talk about the various forms of training, and how to keep it fun. We'll cover the basic body capabilities that a good training program should build and offer some practical guidelines. We'll go into strength training in some detail because we think this is an important area that is often neglected. We'll close with a balanced conditioning program designed by Leslie Spencer, LAT, based on the principles of this chapter and her knowledge and experience working with all levels of gymnasts, from beginners to Olympic contenders.

But first, let's start with advice for parents. If you are a gymnast reading this, hand the book over for a few minutes!

TIPS FOR PARENTS

How old should your child be before getting into gymnastics? Bela Karolyi starts kids at the age of two or three with a program called

"Mom and Me." So the answer is, it's almost never too soon.

And how much time should kids spend in gymnastics? That varies all across the board too. Some kids take classes at the Y once or twice a week for an hour or so. Others are serious about competing and spend part of every day working out with a team. Elite gymnasts spend six to eight hours a day in practice, six days a week! The choice is really up to the gymnast—we are strongly opposed to coercing kids into doing something they don't want to do. Requiring children to practice more than they are willing can be a great way to ruin the sport for them.

What about injuries? According to the statistics, injury rate increases with the competitive level of the gymnast. The injury rate for non-competitive gymnasts is much lower (0.04 percent to 0.07 percent) than the rate reported for beginning competitors (0.7 percent). For advanced gymnasts, the rate is much higher (5.3 percent). Other data indicate that gymnasts in USGF Class I (the highest level) have an injury rate five times that of Class II, 11 times that of Class III, and 25 times that of Class IV.[8]

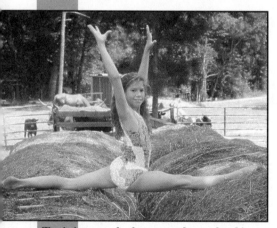

Training can be fun—as shown by this young gymnast at Bela Karolyi's summer camp.

Advanced gymnasts are more likely to get injured because they spend more time in practice and attempt more difficult skills. Time spent in competition seems to be the most dangerous—perhaps because the gymnasts "go for broke."

It is not possible to eliminate all danger from any sport, any more than it is possible to eliminate danger from life.

As parents, you should take an interest in the training program your child gets involved with. Every gymnastics coach has his or her own ideas about creating good gymnasts, and programs can vary dramatically. Some will be harder, some easier, some safer and some more prone to injuries.

Coaches have varying levels of knowledge about conditioning. Most are real experts in their sports, but some coaches may not have equal expertise in exercise physiology. Because they succeed by being single-minded about performance, their plans and programs can sometimes outstrip the capabilities of the gymnast's body.

This chapter gives safe guidelines for training, along with the medical reasons behind our recommendations. The science of sports medicine and exercise physiology has come a long way in the last ten years. Some forms of exercise that were common in the seventies and eighties (deep knee bends and bouncing stretches, for example) are now widely recognized as not only unproductive but unsafe.

As a parent, you should be knowledgeable about the concepts in this chapter and about the conditioning program developed by your child's coach. You can be a big help in keeping your child fit and healthy!

Now you can give the book back!

GETTING MORE BY DOING LESS

You've heard it before: "No pain, no gain."

Don't believe it. One of the great misconceptions in gymnastics and most other sports is that you have to work hard in every exercise, every day. It's probably part of the old Puritan ethic that says that only bad-tasting medicines can cure you.

Forget it. If you work really hard every day, you can look forward to feeling tired all the time, feeling sore all the time, and probably racking up some overuse injuries.

Catabolism and Anabolism: Partners in Growth

Now, you ask, what are the reasons behind the above point of view?

Let me start by talking about two processes that take place in your body: "catabolism" and "anabolism." Once you understand how these work, you'll have a much healthier approach to training.

Catabolism comes from the Greek *kata* meaning "down" and *ballein*, "to throw." Catabolism is a destructive mechanism, a "throwing down" that transforms living tissue to waste products.

When you push a muscle to its limits, you not only deplete its stored energy reserves, you also cause microscopic tears. Those tears must be repaired, and repair work creates waste, so this is a catabolic process.

For example, imagine that a stone crashes through your living room window. It may only leave a small hole, but to repair the window, you have to remove what's left of the glass. That's a lot of broken glass to get rid of.

Fortunately, the other effect of those microscopic muscle tears is to challenge the muscle to rebuild itself to be stronger. If you know someone is going to throw a stone at your window every day, you'll put in quarter-inch safety-glass instead of a fragile eighth-inch sheet. In the same way, the challenged muscle beefs up, which is an anabolic process.

Anabolic comes from the Greek *anabole*, which means "rising up." That's where anabolic steroids get their name, as hormones that build muscle. (That sounds great, except that synthetic anabolic steroids have side effects like liver cancer, sterility and baldness—in both males and females!)

The other effect of hard work on a muscle is that it uses up all the glycogen the muscle has stored for energy. You tear down a muscle's energy reserves (catabolism), so you must allow time to rebuild those reserves (anabolism).

Life is a constant flux of catabolism and anabolism—down with the old, up with the new. The important point is that anabolism takes time. If you exercise the same muscle really hard every day, you don't allow time for the muscle to rebuild and restore its energy. That muscle will be sore and tired all the time. Yes, it will slowly get stronger (because you're young and have incredible resources), but it will be a constant struggle.

Why make training so difficult? Give that muscle a break! Alternate challenge and rest, so the muscle has time to respond to the challenge. Allow anabolism a chance to repair tissue, rebuild reserves, and increase the capacity of the muscle.

In other words, *you should get in shape faster if you let your body breathe a bit!*

Five Kinds of Conditioning

Just about any sport has elements of five kinds of conditioning: strength, endurance, flexibility, coordination and plyometrics.

Strength applies mostly to muscles, although tendons and ligaments also become stronger under a good training program. Endurance really means aerobic fitness and has a lot to do with the condition of the heart, lungs and circulatory system. Flexibility relates to the muscles' ability to stretch and to the elasticity of the tendons and ligaments. As we discussed in the chapter on Body Types, flexibility depends heavily on inheriting good genes from your parents, but your training program can also help. Coordination is your ability to perform the routines. Finally, plyometrics refers to your ability to land and explode upward again, a critical skill for floor routines.

Practical Guidelines for Muscle Conditioning

There are two basic rules:

■ *Alternate days of hard and easy exercise.* You can apply this to specific muscle groups. If you spend hours one day working on landings where your quads, knees and ankles really take a beating, spend the next day concentrating your upper body and give those lower-body landing parts a rest.

■ *Develop opposing muscle groups equally.* For example, gymnasts require Macho Quads, so they spend lots of time developing them. Yet often the hamstrings receive scant attention. This imbalance can cause injuries when weak hamstrings can't keep up with overdeveloped quadriceps. We'll have more to say about this in the section on strength training.

Practical Guidelines for Aerobic Conditioning

The general guideline about rest time also holds true for aerobic conditioning. You will gain faster if you don't overdo it. Here again we have two basic rules:

■ *Work out at 60 percent to 80 percent of your maximum heart rate.* The lower rate may be more effective than a higher rate, because the high rate comes close to being anaerobic. To find your maximum heart rate, subtract your age from 220. Then multiply that by .8 to get your maximum exercise rate. You should keep your pulse under that number. Linda swears by the "talk test," based on years as a Jazzercise groupie: "If you can't jazz and talk at the same time, you're working too hard."

■ *Take time off.* Aerobic conditioning three to five times a week should be plenty. You need the rest of the time for all the anabolism required.

Aerobic conditioning requires extensive anabolism: The heart must become bigger and stronger. The lungs must

72

increase their capacity. The bone marrow must crank out more red blood cells to carry oxygen. Miles of additional capillaries must thread their way into muscles to increase the supply of energy and oxygen. And the whole metabolism must change to a system that burns food for energy instead of dumping it into fat reserves for a future famine.

All of this takes time.

I'm sure you know people who have joined an aerobics class as part of a New Year's resolution. They go three times a week for six weeks, and each time it's the same—grunts and struggles. If the class aims at people already in good shape, the new folks are in real trouble! Sore, tired. . .where, they wonder, are all the benefits aerobics is supposed to offer? At the end of the class six weeks later, they quit.

The irony is that six weeks is about the amount of time the body takes to respond to the challenge! Just when their bodies are becoming capable of enjoying the workout and really benefitting, these folks throw in the towel.

The moral of all this is that it takes time to get in condition. You cannot substitute extra-hard work for time; in fact, extra-hard work only makes things worse. Use the idea of anabolic rest to guide you when you start something new or decide to increase your workout. You'll progress faster by taking it a little easy on the alternate day. (Have you noticed that we keep repeating this? We want to penetrate the consciousness of all you compulsive types out there!)

Practical Guidelines for Flexibility Training

How, you may wonder, are we going to tell you to get more by doing less here? Stretching exercises are extremely important, and they should be done frequently—before, during and after workout. Do *not* get slack about stretching!

Why is stretching so important? It prevents injury, *and* it prevents pain. If you get stiff and sore from workouts, it's because you skimped on stretching. You will be amazed at how much difference stretching can make in how you feel, not to mention how flexible you are.

The key here is how you stretch. Depending on how you do it, stretching can increase flexibility and make you feel better—or tighten you up and make you hurt more. Stretching can prevent injuries or promote them.

- *Static stretches promote flexibility and prevent injuries.* A static stretch is one where you go into the stretch gradually and hold it for six to 30 seconds. *No bouncing!* If your muscles start burning, relax a bit and give the blood a chance to circulate. Then resume.

- *Dynamic stretches promote tightness and may cause injuries.* Dynamic stretches are those where you are constantly moving—swinging from side to side or bouncing. We don't see a use for this kind of stretch in improving flexibility. It is a conditioning exercise that you should do only after you warm up.

Dynamic stretches don't help you gain flexibility, and they can cause injuries. Here's why: As you probably know (if you don't know, see the chapter on Body Basics), muscles connect to bones by means of tendons. At the place where each muscle joins its tendon, there are "Golgi tendon organs" embedded in the muscle. The Golgi organs are tiny stretch receptors—under a microscope, they look like little springs. When they get yanked too hard or too quickly, they send out a signal that makes the muscle *contract*!

The Golgi organs are a protective mechanism: They try to prevent muscle tears by contracting the muscle. Obviously, if you're trying to gain flexibility by lengthening and stretching your muscles, the one thing you *don't* want to happen is a mass attack of the Golgi tendon organs. Yet this is exactly what dynamic stretches invite. When a stretch is too quick (any time a stretch is quick at all), the Golgi organs tell the muscle to contract.

So you are trying to stretch, and your muscle is trying to contract. It's a pitched battle: The harder you try, the more you bounce, the worse it gets. It does not help your flexibility. Sometimes the muscle responds to the Golgi organs so strongly that you get a muscle spasm—a "charley horse" in the hamstrings is one common example.

The way to avoid automatic contraction from stretching is to stretch slowly, and hold it. Give those Golgi guys time to relax. You'll be more flexible, and more fit too.

Practical Guidelines for Coordination Training

Rotate through different gymnastic routines: floor work today, bars tomorrow, vault the next day, and so on. Don't practice the same skills two days in a row. This is really a form of cross-training, and you'll find that each practice adds to the others. We commonly see a situation where a gymnast works all day on a particular release without making much progress. After spending the next several days on totally different activities, the gymnast comes back to the release and viola! There it is. Muscles, like the mind, seem to have a form of subconscious activity that goes on even when they aren't working actively on a particular skill.

Your ability as a gymnast will increase much faster by continually varying your workouts than if you worked on each skill for days or weeks before rotating.

Can you imagine trying to become a concert pianist by playing only one piece? No. Keep your routines varied, work all your muscles equally, and you'll have a synergism going for you that will make you a better gymnast—and training more fun!

Practical Guidelines for Plyometrics Training

We usually think of strengthening muscles by contracting them. But in plyometrics, muscles gain power by

75

being dynamically stretched. A typical plyometric conditioning routine is to jump from a sturdy platform to the mat and immediately leap up again as high as possible. (The height of the platform would depend on your physical condition.) This trains your leg muscles to store energy as they lengthen during the landing, and then release that energy as you leap up.

As you might imagine, plyometric conditioning can easily lead to injuries if you do it wrong. It's like taking dynamic stretching (which we told you not to do as part of flexibility conditioning) and making it super-dynamic. Before plyometric exercises, you should warm up thoroughly, and you should *always* do these exercises under supervision. The best supervisor is your coach or an athletic trainer who can devise the right program based on your age, weight and physical condition.

Cross Training

Now we want to come back to fun. We talked about varying your gymnastics routines to provide rest. Another result of changing things often is that it makes training more fun, too.

And you can gain some extra benefits by working out in other sports. Try running, swimming, cycling, strength training. All of these can be great ways to increase strength, gain coordination and improve aerobic fitness, and they keep life more interesting.

If possible, do some of your running and cycling on real roads instead of on a treadmill or an exercise bike. When you run or cycle on a real road or track, you must constantly compensate for uneven ground and maintain your balance. This works a whole raft of small muscles that are important in gymnastics.

Be aware that running is a two-edged sword: It strengthens knees, but the pounding of too much running can cause stress fractures in the tibia.

GETTING STRONGER

Here we talk about strength training. Before you girls skip this chapter because "girl gymnasts don't need to be strong," stay tuned long enough to illuminate your minds about a few misconceptions.

Misconceptions About Strength Training

Misconception #1: "Strength training is just another term for weight lifting."
Wrong. The object of weight lifting is to lift weights. (Or maybe to build bulging muscles that impress girls at the beach.) The object of strength training is to build strength, to enhance your gymnastics performance and to prevent injuries.

The American Orthopaedic Society for Sports Medicine defines strength training as "The use of progressive resistance methods (which includes using body weight, free weights and machines) to increase one's ability to exert or resist force."[9] In gymnastics, strength training gives you the ability to resist the force of gravity!

Misconception #2: "Girls don't have to be strong."
Wrong. Dr. Jensen thinks one reason there are so many shoulder and wrist problems in female gymnasts is that they ignore upper body strength training. The guys do routines that obviously require strong arms and shoulders, but gals can also benefit from a tougher upper body. For one thing, it makes the routines *easier*.

Maybe you're worried that if you develop strong arms and shoulders you'll bulk up like one of those oil-covered females on the cover of some body-building magazine. Not so—for one thing, you don't have the hormones for it. It takes testosterone to make muscles bulge. Secondly, you won't be lifting big weights several hours a day; instead, you'll be moving small weights to build just the strength you need for gymnastics.

It *is* possible to be strong and beautiful at the same time.

Misconception #3: "Strength training doesn't work for kids."

This has been a matter of some dispute in the medical profession. However, recent studies show that muscle strength in children does increase with strength training.[10] In one study, a group of 18 pre-adolescent children did strength training three times a week for nine weeks and on average increased their strength by more than 40 percent. Another study showed that kids could increase grip, flexed arm hang, pull-ups *and* flexibility with strength training. Still other studies demonstrate that strength training can increase measurable quantities like the vertical jump. Dr. Jensen and Leslie Spencer have no doubts that strength training can also increase gymnastic performance.

Misconception #4: "Strength training kills flexibility."

Not so! The same medical article referenced above also reports that kids maintain their flexibility easily, so long as general flexibility exercises are part of the exercise program. It even appears that strength training can *improve* flexibility!

Misconception #5: "Strength training isn't safe for kids."

The risk of injury is extremely low in a properly designed and supervised program. Obviously, if a little kid tries to bench-press 150 pounds, something's going to give, and it won't be the weight. Lifting heavy weights can be very dangerous for kids—*Don't do it* until you're well into puberty.

In contrast, low weights and a high number of repetitions is extremely safe. And this kind of training also helps prevent other injuries.[11] Animal studies show that strength training can also increase the strength of bones and ligaments.[12]

78

Agonist and Antagonist

This is an important concept in strength training: the development of equal strength in opposing muscles. For every movement there's at least one agonist muscle (agonist comes from the Greek *agonistes*, "one who contends for a prize"). Opposing each agonist is an antagonist muscle, which works to the opposite effect. For example, when you curl a weight, the biceps muscle is the agonist and the triceps is the antagonist; when you squat, the quadriceps is the agonist and the hamstring the antagonist.

Both agonist and antagonist muscles should have equal strength, or muscle imbalance results. This can lead to muscle strains and other injuries.

Types of Strength Training

Strength training is by definition "resistance training," and there are many ways for a muscle to work against resistance. For the three general categories, we go back to the Greeks:

Isometric exercise
Isometric comes from the Greek words *isos* meaning "equal" and *metron*, "measure." In isometric exercises, the joint doesn't move. If you hold your leg out in front of you and contract all the muscles, you're doing an isometric strengthening exercise. Each muscle is working against its opposing muscle, and both become stronger. You can also do isometric exercises with weights or machines, by keeping the weight or machine in one position and working against the resistance without moving.

Isometric exercises are particularly useful during rehabilitation, when you want to provide muscle conditioning without stressing the joint.

Isotonic exercise

"Tonic" comes from the Greek word tonos, meaning tone or tension. In isotonic exercises you use free weights or machines that move the joint through its full range. This is the kind of strength training we're all most familiar with.

Isokinetic exercise

This is a new form of strength training that requires some fairly exotic machines. "Kinetic" comes from the Greek verb *kinein*, meaning "to move," and isokinetic machines limit the speed of motion. You set the machine on a speed and that's the maximum speed the machine will move. Then you see how much torque or power you can develop against that speed. It's a good way to measure the capability of the muscle. It's also a specific tool for tailoring exercise to either fast-twitch or slow-twitch muscles. (See the chapter on Body Types for an explanation of twitches.)

Varieties of Isotonic Experience

As we said, isotonic exercises are the most common form of strength training. These, too, come in several flavors:

Free weights

Free weights are barbells of varying weights. They have some advantages and disadvantages. The advantages are that, like riding a bicycle on a real road instead of using an exercise bicycle, free weights use more muscles. Along with the main muscle you're working, a host of other muscles comes into play to keep everything on track.

The disadvantage of free weights is linked to the advantage: Free weights require much more supervision and training for correct use. To keep the exercise safe and get the most benefit, you should use each weight in a very exact and specific way. Free weights are easy to use incorrectly.

Stacked weight machines

Stacked weight machines are the simplest form of machine and have been around a long time, as evidenced by the rusty contraptions moldering in the back rooms of many gyms and community centers. These machines use (not surprisingly) stacks of metal weights and various pulleys, and they solve some of the problems of free weights by limiting motion to certain directions. However, you still require education and supervision to use stacked weights correctly.

Constant resistance machines

Here's the type made famous by Nautilus®. Using cams and other clever mechanisms, these machines provide constant resistance throughout the range of motion, something that simple stacked-weight machines don't do. (We could explain why—it has to do with vectors and so forth—but we'll spare you.)

The other advantage offered by machines is that they position your body so that only one motion is possible. While this limits the number of muscles worked by any one machine, it does ensure that the correct muscles are being worked. So you don't need as much supervision when you use these machines.

By the way, the name Nautilus comes from the spiral seashell you may be familiar with. This is the same shape of the cams that provide the constant resistance. (A bit of trivia for your collection.)

Fluid resistance machines

These are sometimes called "hydrofitness" machines, because they use pistons that travel through fluid-filled chambers. The fluid gives constant resistance, and it also absorbs shocks, a nice feature.

Rubber bands

Let's not forget the low-tech approach, which can be an ideal way to exercise certain muscle groups like the rotator cuff, for example. There are many forms of stretchable bands, and many ways to use them. Once again, this takes some supervision, but bands tend to be a very safe form of resistance training.

General Guidelines for Strength Training

Several factors are important in making strength training safe and productive for pre-adolescent gymnasts:

Pre-participation history and physical
Your doctor should look for any health problems that might predispose you to injury. He or she should also check your flexibility and range-of-motion to make sure there are no problems there that strength training could worsen.

Warmup and cool-down periods
Before you start a strength training workout, you should warm up with slow jogging or stationary bike riding for five to ten minutes. Then spend a few minutes with stretches.

After your resistance routine, slow down with a few minutes of jogging, followed by stretching. Be sure to stretch all the muscles you've worked—otherwise they will tend to tighten up. Stretching helps oxygen get back into the muscles and it maintains flexibility.

If strength training is part of an entire workout schedule, it should come after warmup and before stretching.

Length and frequency of sessions
Strength training should not last longer than one hour maximum, and should be done approximately three times a week (never two days in a row). Remember what we said about rest time?

How hard?

It depends. Here is a table we have adapted from the previous referenced article by Wolohan and Michell:[13]

Guidelines for a gymnastic strength-training program.

Ages	Maximum weight * (resistance)	Number of exercises per body part**	Number of repetitions	Number of sets
0-9	None	0	0	0
9-11	Very light	1	12-15	2
12-14	Light	1	10-12	3
15-16	Moderate	2	7-11	3-4
17+	Heavy	>2	6-10	4-6

* The trainer should determine the amount of weight a gymnast can move through a complete range of motion. "Very light" is less than 30 percent of the one-repetition maximum (RM); "Light" is less than 50 percent of one RM; "Moderate", 70 percent; and heavy, 80 percent.
** A total-body weight-training program that concentrates on the large muscles is best.
*** Note that repetitions can be increased somewhat *if the amount of weight is reduced.* Fewer reps of more weight tend to increase strength and bulk. More reps of lower weight tend to increase strength and endurance.

[8] Pettrone FA, Ricciardelli E.: Gymnastics Injuries: The Virginia Experience. *Am J Sports Med* 15:59-62, 1987.

[9] Cahill BR, moderator and ed. Proceedings of the Conference on Strength Training and the Prepubescent, Chicago, Ill: American Orthopaedic Society for Sports Medicine; 1988:3.

[10] Wolohan, MJ, Michell, LJ. Strength training in children. *The Journal of Musculoskeletal Medicine* 1990; 7(7): 37-52.

[11] Micheli LJ. The exercising child: injuries, Pediatric Exercise Science. 1989;1(4): 329-336 and Duda M. Prepubescent strength training gains support, *Physical Sports-Medicine;* 1988:3.

[12] Tipton CM, Matthes RD, Maynard JA, et al. The influence of physical activity on ligaments and tendons. *Medical Science Sports Exercise.* 1975;7(3): 165-175.

[13] Wolohan, MJ, Michell, LJ. Strength training in children. *The Journal of Musculoskeletal Medicine* 1990; 7(7): 37-52.

A BALANCED CONDITIONING PROGRAM

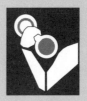

We include here warmup routines, stretches and conditioning exercises for novice to advanced gymnasts. Complete training programs for all levels of gymnasts could easily fill an entire book, so this section is necessarily shorter than that. However, it will give you a good basic program to build upon.

Warmup

Start your workouts with a gentle warmup—easy running for ten minutes or so. Run different ways: with your knees up, on your toes (heels up), with straight legs forward, and then with straight legs backwards. Skip while you circle your arms.

The idea is to get the blood moving and loosen up before you place any major stresses on your body.

85

Stretches

After warmup, be sure to stretch out all your major muscle groups. This will help increase your flexibility; even more important, it will help prevent injuries. Do stretches slowly, easing into them, and *don't bounce.* Unless instructed otherwise, *hold* each stretch at least six seconds—preferably 30 seconds.

We'll start at the top with standing stretches.

Neck Stretch

Roll head gently and slowly forward and backward,
then side to side (bending neck).
Then look side to side (twisting neck).
Then circle head clockwise and counterclockwise.
Repeat several times. ■

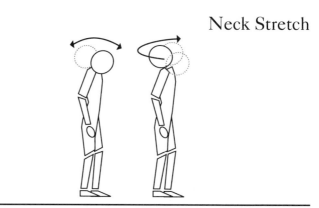

Calf Stretch

Lean against a wall with one leg behind and heel down. With leg straight, press hips into the wall.

Maintain above stretch while bending knee of rear leg. You should feel stretch move down into heel. ■

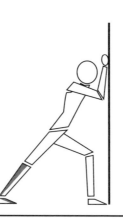
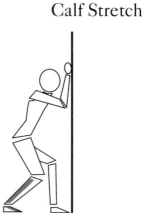

Quad Stretch

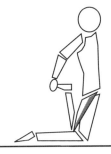

Kneel with back straight. Hold one foot, push hip forward and pull ankle toward your body. Standing, this is also a good balance exercise. ◼

Hamstring Stretch

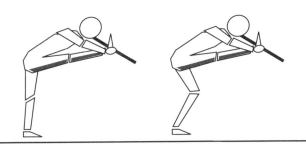

Place heel on waist-high object. Keep back straight and bend nose to knee. To increase stretch, bend knee of standing leg. ◼

Shoulder Stretches

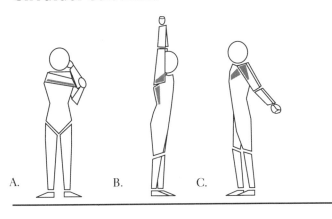

A.   B.   C.

A. Grab elbow with other hand and pull arm gently across body. Repeat on other side.
B. Pull both arms above and behind head, keeping elbows straight.
C. Grasp hands behind your back. Press arms up, keeping back and elbows straight. ◼

Arm Windmills

Holding arms straight out from sides, move them slowly in big circles, forwards and backwards. Keep elbows straight. ■

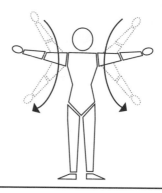

Wrist Flexor and Extensor Stretch

Use one hand to stretch the other wrist forwards and backwards. Do this various ways: arm straight, arm bent, palm up and palm down. ■

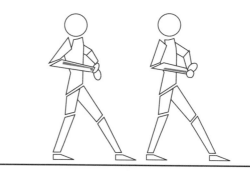

Trunk Stretches

A. Lying on back, pull both legs and head into tight ball.
B. Extend legs and arms over head.
C. In sitting position, cross one leg over the other and twist body toward the raised leg. ■

A.

B.

C.

Groin Stretches

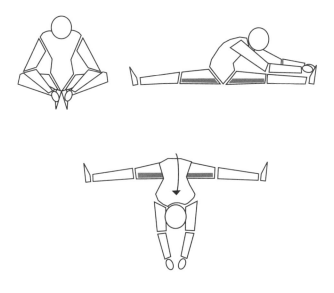

A. Sit with legs in long diamond in front of you and lean forward. This stretches groin and gluteus maximus.
B. Sit with legs in short diamond (feet close to body, heels together). Lean forward with straight back and press down on knees to stretch groin and inner thigh.
C. With legs straight to sides, bend right ear to right knee. Repeat on left.
D. With legs straight to the side, lean forward and press chest to floor. To provide additional stretch for mid-back, rotate upper body to left and right. ■

Ankle Rolls

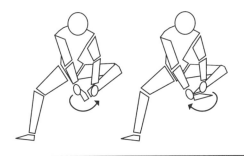

Sitting down, use hands to roll ankles and stretch in all directions. ■

89

Strengthening Exercises

These exercises will help you increase the strength of important muscle groups. Do them after you are warmed up. Carry out these exercises according to the guidelines in the previous section. The general rule is "up fast, down slow."

Wrist Rotation

Use a weight that allows 20-30 repetitions.
A. With palm up, raise and lower the weight to strengthen the wrist flexor muscles.
B. Do same exercise with palm down to strengthen the wrist extensor muscles.
C. Stabilize elbow on table with forearm and wrist off the edge. Turn wrist left and right, as if turning a door handle. ■

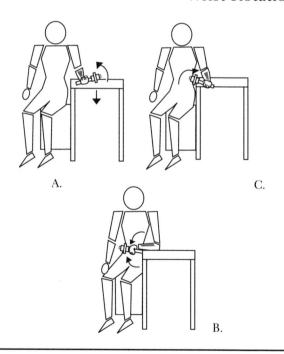

A.

C.

B.

Pushups on Parallel Bars

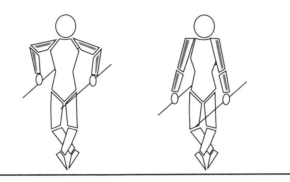

Suspend yourself from parallel bars. Push up until elbows are straight; then go down until elbows bend at 90°. ■

Quadriceps Wall Sit

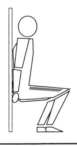

Leaning against a wall, slide down until in a sitting position, thighs parallel to floor and lower legs straight up and down. Hold this position 10-20 seconds. ■

With appropriate weight on ankle, lift lower leg behind you. Repeat on other side. ∎

Hamstring Curls

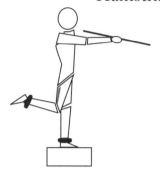

A. With knees straight and weight on ankle, lift entire leg behind you. Repeat on other side.
B. To balance muscles, lift entire leg in front of you, toes toward the ceiling. Repeat on other side.∎

Hip Flexor/Extensor

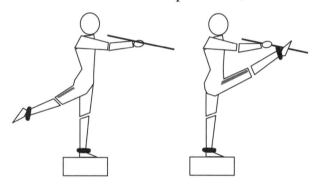

A. With stretch-able band on ankle, pull leg across in front, keeping leg and back straight. Repeat on other side.
B. To balance muscles, pull straight leg out to side, away from centerline of body. Repeat on other side.∎

Hip Adduction and Abduction

A.

B.

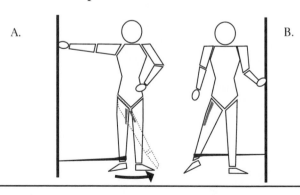

Hip Extension

With legs extended
over edge of table,
raise legs until back
is straight and legs
are parallel to floor.
Do not arch back. ■

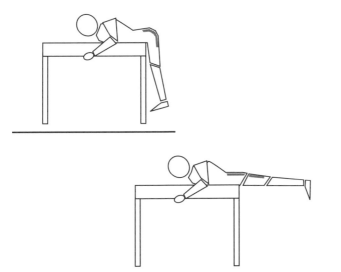

Back Extension

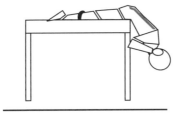

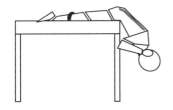

With upper body
extended over
edge of table, raise
body until back
is straight and
parallel with floor.
Do not arch back! ■

93

Bridges

Get into backbend
and push hands
and heels together.
Hold, back off
and repeat. ■

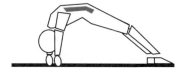

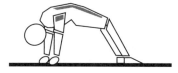

Arch-ups

Lie on one side
on mat. Without
pushing up with
arms, arch right
shoulder and hip
toward each
other. Repeat on
other side. ■

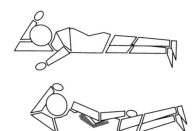

Abdominal Workout

A. Lie on back with knees bent. With arms in front, curl upper body toward knees. Works upper abdominals (abdominus rectus).

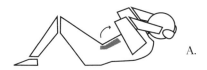

A.

B. Lift and twist trunk alternately to right and left; aim right elbow at left knee and left elbow at right knee. Works obliques.

B.

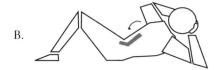

C. Reverse crunch: Important exercise for the lower back! Keep legs tucked and lift pelvis off floor. *Do not* swing legs. A very small movement (one to two inches) to be done *slowly*. ∎

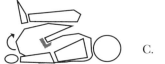

C.

Advanced Strengthening Exercises

These moves are not easy—don't attempt them unless you have some experience and can do at least one repetition fairly easily.

V-ups on Bars

Hang from parallel bars, legs down and toes pointed. Keeping legs straight and toes pointed, bring knees up to nose and then lower. ■

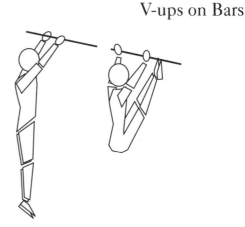

Press Handstand

Press into a handstand. Bring legs down keeping knees straight and swing legs around arms until feet are in front. Only hands should touch the floor. Repeat.■

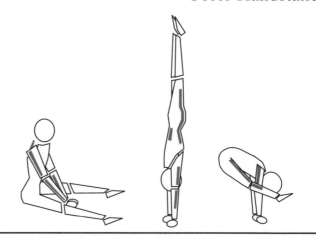

Handstand Pushup

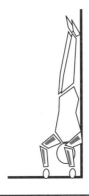 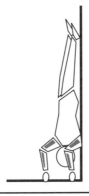

Using a wall to help stability, push up from headstand into handstand. Keep back straight at all times and *Do not arch!* Push up until elbows are straight, then lower until elbow is bent almost halfway. Repeat. ■

Tic-Tocs

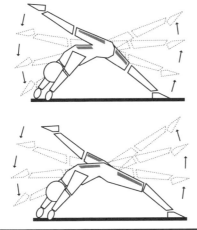

From a backbend, kick right leg over until foot touches floor, then return to backbend position. Repeat on other side. ■

Hollow Rocks

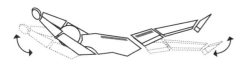

Keep legs and arms straight and abdominal muscles tight. Rock back and forth without touching head, hands or feet to ground. ■

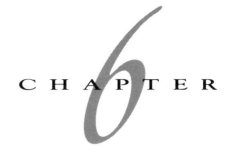

CHAPTER

The Spine

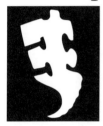

"Hip bone connected to the thigh bone" is pretty simple, but "spine bone connected to the spine bone" is not. What an intricate and clever system to keep our front legs off the ground!

As the only animals walking around upright, we humans sometimes pay a price in back pain. Gymnasts are particularly vulnerable because of the incredible stress their spines absorb. Nature has provided a unique system designed to keep everybody up straight, and there go those gymnasts, tying their backs in knots.

As a result, the trunk and spine account for about 12-19 percent of reported injuries.[14] Competition gymnasts suffer about five times as much lower-back injury as comparable non-athletes.[15] The rate of reinjury is alarming, too, especially in elite gymnasts with heavy competitive schedules. We think most reinjury could be avoided by complete rehabilitation before returning to full activity. Yes, you can get by and even perform with an injured back, but do you want to spend your entire life with a spine that's already 80 years old when you are only 20?

Fortunately, most young people don't get injured because they have very flexible ligaments and very soft and forgiving discs between their vertebrae. Most of the time, you gymnasts can get away with stuff the rest of us wouldn't even attempt: the ultimate swayback (hyperextension) and nose-to-the-floor (hyperflexion).

As you get older, your discs gradually dry out and become less rubbery, and you lose some of your ability to hyper-extend and flex. That's why you'll never see a 30-year-old "comeback" gymnast at the Olympics!

Because young backs are so resilient, most back injuries to gymnasts are simple sprains and strains that go away in a week or two. If you get a back pain that does *not* go away quickly, *go to a doctor!* Don't let anyone call you a wimp for complaining about low back pain. Any back pain lasting more than two weeks calls for a complete evaluation by a doctor, including history and physical. The doctor should also take back x-rays from five different angles, and perhaps even bone scans.

But before we get too specific about injuries, let's see how the spine works.

SPINAL ANATOMY: NATURE'S NO-OPEN ZIPPER

The cartoon idea of a spine is a stack of disks, with a hole in the center for the spinal cord and pointy things on the back side like spines on a dinosaur. Well, it's a bit more complex— more like two side-by-side zippers designed never to open.

The Individual Vertebra

The drawing to the right shows a single vertebra. This particular vertebra is from the lower (lumbar) portion of your back where most back problems occur. Looking closer, we see. . .

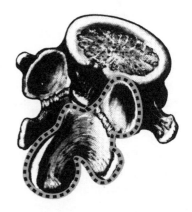

Lumbar vertebra, showing major elements.

100

The vertebral body

This is the round job that holds up most of the weight. A rubbery disc sits between the vertebral bodies to absorb shock and allow the spine to bend. Without the discs, the spine would bend very little and it would be as fragile as a stack of children's building blocks.

The disc uses the jelly doughnut idea. The outside is a tough fibrous material (actually, it's quite a bit tougher than the outside of a jelly doughnut), and the inside is a thick, shock-absorbing jelly.

The spinal canal

Right behind the vertebral body is the spinal canal, the protective tunnel that encases your spinal cord. The spinal cord is where all the nerves from your body come together to travel up to your brain and back again. Nerves join the spinal cord all along its length.

We all know that the cells of the body are so small, they can only be seen through a microscope. But did you know that some nerve cells are several feet long? Of course, they're very skinny, so you still need a microscope.

In greatly simplified terms, the length of the nerve carries electrical messages from your brain to your muscles, and from your sense organs (taste, touch, smell, etc.) to your brain. In a way, the nerves in the spinal canal are like the railroad tracks of a subway, carrying messages like subway cars.

If you break a vertebral body and it cuts through the spinal cord, you break the track, and the break is permanent. The cars don't get through, and the muscles connected to those nerves end up paralyzed. A break high in the neck will paralyze most of the body, where a break in the lumbar region lower down will paralyze only the legs.

Well, let's not get depressing about paralysis. That kind of injury is *extremely* rare in gymnastics!

The processes

Here we are talking about the superior and inferior *articular processes* and the *spinous process*. Whew, what a mouthful. "Superior" is the fancy medical term meaning that it's on top, while "inferior" means that it's on the bottom. One is not better or worse that the other!

Here's where the permanent zippers come in: Along each side of the spine, every *superior process* has a shallow socket that an *inferior process* can fit into. So each *superior process* of one vertebra holds the *inferior process* of the vertebra above it, and so on, all up and down the spine. It's like two zippers, one on each side, each zipper held together by ligaments and muscles. They move enough to give you the flexibility to bend and twist, but not enough to let the spine come apart!

The *transverse processes* and the *spinous processes* provide additional places where muscles and ligaments attach to control and stabilize the spine. There are *lots* of little (and big) muscles, and we'll spare you by not naming them.

The pars interarticularis and the Scotty-dog fracture

Why are we naming something so unpronounceable? Sorry. The spine has quite a few long names associated with it, at least one of which is worse than this one. The reason for naming this place is that it is a region that can get damaged during gymnastics.

Look back at the drawing of the lumbar vertebra—do you see the outline of a little Scotty dog? He (or she) is facing to the right: The *spinous process* and *inferior articular process* are legs, and the superior articular process is the head. A break of the *pars interarticularis* looks like a collar around the dog's neck, and it's often called a "Scotty-dog fracture."

We'll have more to say about this later.

The Spinal Column

The drawing shows the five parts of the spine, with a total of 33 vertebrae.

The various types of vertebrae look a bit different from each other because they do different jobs.

The seven cervical vertebrae are designed to keep your head firmly attached but easily movable. Did you know you have the same number of neck vertebrae as a giraffe?

The 12 thoracic vertebrae come equipped with handy attachment points for the 12 pairs of ribs, so they allow relatively little movement. You wouldn't want your ribs all sticking out at different angles.

Most of the twisting your back can do comes courtesy of the five lumbar vertebrae. These vertebrae also take the most punishment from gymnastics and from life in general. You don't hear many people complaining of upper back pain, but you hear plenty of groaning about lower back pain. Neck pain, too. Also pains in the neck, but that's different.

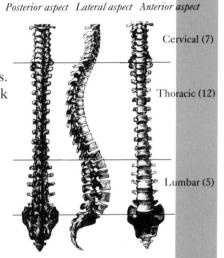

Posterior aspect   Lateral aspect   Anterior aspect

Cervical (7)

Thoracic (12)

Lumbar (5)

The spinal column.

The sacrum looks like a giant curved arrowhead pointing downward. Actually, it's five vertebrae that fuse together to form the back side of the pelvis. Hanging from the end of the sacrum is the coccyx, a collection of four or five small fused vertebrae. This is the "tailbone," and you'll only know you have one if you land on it too hard!

Holding It Up

We talked about the muscles on the back side of the vertebrae, which help hold the whole contraption together.

Naturally, there are muscles all up and down the front side as well. The most important are the *iliopsoas* muscles that tie the lumbar vertebrae to the pelvis and the upper part of the femur. These muscles help you raise your leg and do sit-ups.

Equally important in stabilizing the back are the abdominal muscles!

I'm sure you're familiar with radio towers in rural areas—those tall, skinny metal structures with lights to warn nearby aircraft. If you look closely, you'll see thin guy wires anchoring the tower to the ground. Wires come from the top and sides of the tower and attach to the ground some distance away. Without those wires, the tower would come crashing down at the first breeze.

The abdominal muscles do the same thing for the spine. They aren't close to the spine, but they're very important!

There are three main abdominal muscles: *internal obliques, external obliques* and *rectus abdominus*. The two sets of obliques slant in opposite directions, while the *rectus abdominus* runs straight up and down (that's the one that has the neat rippled look when you really get in shape). All three muscles work like nature's version of the bias-ply tire, keeping the internal organs neatly in place and stabilizing the back.

You don't have to remember all these details, but you should remember that there are two sides to the back, and one of them is the front!

If you remove the guy wires from one side of that radio tower, it will collapse. The same is true of your back: If your abdominals are weak, you are much more likely to have back trouble. The best exercises for your back are upper-body and lower-body curl-ups. Shape up those wimpy abs!

By the way, one reason overweight people are prone to back problems—especially men with "beer guts"—is that the abdominals have to go around curves to do their jobs. Plus, the center of gravity shifts forward and increases the leverage on the spine. Not a pretty picture, in more ways than one.

Preventing Injury

Too often, the importance of a strong back goes unrecognized in gymnastics. People worry about flexible backs, without enough attention to increasing strength. You can be both flexible and strong, and you should be. Think about it—all your other limbs attach to your trunk, and they all rely on the strength of the back.

Be especially aware of your back when changing training routines. Perhaps you move up to a higher level of performance, or you move to a tougher gym, or you start working out more. Don't jump into anything new too suddenly. Give your body time to adapt, and include plenty of abdominal work to strengthen your back.

The second important point is to include extensive static stretching routines in your warmup. Stretch your back and neck muscles slowly and thoroughly—no bouncing!

The third important thing, as we already mentioned, is not to ignore injuries, and to give yourself time for a complete recovery before returning to a full workout.

A strong, well-stretched, healthy back will not only prevent back injury—it will also help prevent injuries in general!

COMMON AND NOT-SO-COMMON BACK PROBLEMS

Most back problems in gymnasts are not serious, even many with serious sounding names, as you'll see. However, back problems should not be ignored! Let us say again, any time you have pain for longer than two weeks, see a doctor.

Sprains and Strains

Because there are so many little muscles and ligaments all crammed together around the spine, it's virtually impossible to separate ligament sprains from muscle strains. Fortunately, it doesn't make any difference.

Causes:

Sprains and strains occur at the extremes of motion— hyperextension, hyperflexion, or too much rotation. You'll be especially likely to get one of these injuries if you don't warm up properly. One good way to injure your back in a hurry is to jump into dynamic bouncing stretches without a good amount of slow static warmup first.

Symptoms:

You'll feel sudden pain and loss of motion. Generally, pain will be localized in one area, and certain motions, either active or passive, will make it worse. Many times, you can feel a sprain or strain two ways: (1) it hurts, and (2) you can feel a lump where the muscle has gone into spasm.

Treatment:

Start with RICE—Rest, Ice, Compression. . .well, we're not sure exactly how to fit in Elevation! Stop using the muscle, apply ice, and if necessary, support the injured part with a back or neck brace. Deep massage at the point of pain can often help relieve muscle spasm and pain.

Once initial pain has subsided (24 to 48 hours), use moist heat, gentle stretching and light isometric exercise. Increase the strength of the muscles with resistance training recommended by your doctor or trainer, using free weights, machines, curl-ups, etc. Remember that one possible reason for the injury was that the muscle wasn't strong enough.

Generally, muscle strain symptoms go away in three to seven days. If pain lasts longer, a ligament sprain may be the culprit—it takes a bit longer to mend. As the ligament heals, it will tend to be stiff, so you will need to continue gentle stretching and range-of-motion exercises. Ultrasound and alternating heat and cold treatments may also be helpful.

See a doctor if this injury results in numbness or tingling in an arm or leg, or if it causes pain that travels down into an arm or leg. This could indicate that a nerve is involved, and this is nothing to fool around with. Also see a doctor if all symptoms do not go away in two weeks.

Curvature of the Spine

Types of curvature:

We mention this topic here, *not* because spines grow into weird shapes when exposed to gymnastics, but because some amount of abnormal curvature is relatively common to the population at large, and gymnasts are no exception. Spinal curvature is not some rare and gruesome affliction that dooms you to living in the moldy corners of Notre Dame and ringing bells.

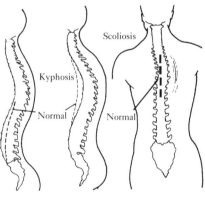

Three types of abnormal spinal curvature.

There are three basic types of curvature: *lordosis* (in common terms, the sway back), *kyphosis* (humped back), and *scoliosis* (a sideways curvature). You may consider scoliosis the worst, but many gymnasts have it. It's nothing unusual.

No one really knows what causes abnormal spinal curvature. In many cases, it seems that the spine just develops a little "off-spec." If you have one of these conditions, it should not hurt your performance as a gymnast, and it should not be painful. However, it should be followed by a doctor, as it may get worse during your adolescent growth spurt.

107

Treatment:

The primary treatment is what you should be doing anyway—plenty of back strengthening exercise. If the problem starts getting worse during adolescence, bracing can help prevent it without scuttling your gymnastics career. If the scoliosis gets severe (which is rare), it may be necessary to have rods or other internal fixation devices surgically implanted. In this case, your gymnastics career may be over, but you can still excel in sports that don't require a super-flexible spine.

Spondylolysis: the Scotty-Dog Stress Fracture

Spondylolysis (spon-dil-o-li-sis) comes from the Greek words *spondylo*, meaning vertebra, and *lysis*, meaning loosening or coming apart. Sounds bad, doesn't it? Actually, it's fairly common, in humans at least. No other animals seem to have it, perhaps because they're not walking around on just two legs.

Remember the drawing of the vertebra and the *pars interarticularis?* (That was the neck of the Scotty dog.) We mentioned that this area can fracture. The most common injury is a stress fracture, called a *pars defect* or *spondylolysis* (official medical terminology) or a Scotty-dog stress fracture (used by cool sports-medicine types).

In some cases, the bone in the pars degrades until fibrous tissue replaces it. You still have a complete vertebra, except that the neck of one (or more) of your Scotty dogs doesn't show up on an x-ray because it isn't bone anymore.

Gymnasts tend to have more spondylolysis than non-athletes: In one study of 100 competitive female gymnasts, 11 percent had spondylolysis, compared to 2.3 percent of an equivalent non-gymnast population.[16] Other athletes at high risk include pole vaulters, hurdlers, and weightlifters—all involved with back-bashing sports.

As you can imagine from the large number of gymnasts with this condition, it is not a crippling problem. Normally, the defect heals, pain goes away, and the gymnast never knows that a tiny bit of back has changed from bone to fibrous tissue.

Causes:

Think back to the drawing of the vertebra. Remember that the big vertebral body carries all the weight. And the little processes have most of the muscle hookups. The *pars interarticularis* is the main support structure that connects one vertebra to another, and much the stress of moving the weight and twisting the spine travels through it.

Gymnasts are prone to pars problems, because they routinely hyperextend and hyperflex the spine (for example, back and front walkovers). Jarring dismounts, vaults and flips also take a toll—gymnasts frequently absorb vertical impact forces up to 11 times their body weight!

Muscular fatigue also seems to play a role. When your muscles are fresh, they absorb stress easily. But as they tire, they pass stress on to tendons and bones. One study reported that gymnastic clubs that practiced 20 to 30 hours a week had significantly higher injury rates than those that practiced only four to six hours a week.[17] Here's one more reason to strengthen your back and not to work out past the point of exhaustion!

Genetic predisposition to injury also seems to play a role, particularly in gymnasts who are naturally swaybacked (lordotic).

Since there's a pars on either side of the spine, they help back each other up. Nevertheless, sometimes the stress is too great, and the pars cracks. One of your Scotty dogs now has a collar.

Symptoms:

Stress fractures may not show symptoms initially, but only as additional damage piles up in an already damaged area. If you have aching lower-back (lumbar) pain that doesn't go away, you could have a Scotty-Dog fracture. Perhaps you first notice a little pain during a back flip or back walkover, perhaps just on one side. Then it becomes worse—it may even interfere with normal activities, like sitting in school. It usually goes away if you lie down for a while, but it's still bothering you several weeks later. All this means that you should *go to a doctor!*

Diagnosis:

One easy test your doctor may do is to have you stand on one leg with the other bent and just off the floor, and then lean back. If that hurts, it may be a pars problem.

Your doctor will probably do x-rays and bone scans if the above test indicates a possible problem. (For more information on diagnostic techniques, see the chapter on Body Basics.)

Treatment:

When bone breaks, the first thing that happens is that the bits of broken bone are reabsorbed by the body. Then new bone is laid down to mend the fracture. It takes about two weeks before new bone starts to fill in the gaps. Then it takes about four more weeks for the process to complete. During this time (six weeks) you should stay away from hyperflexion and hard landings. Instead, work on back conditioning exercises!

If you have a severe problem, your doctor may decide to brace your back. In some cases, nipples-to-knees casts have even been used, although most doctors feel that they offer little or no benefit over simple bracing.

This is potentially a serious long-term problem; however, it can heal or become "asymptomatic" (stop bothering you). *If you take care of it!*

Spondylolisthesis

And you thought it was hard to pronounce *pars interarticularis?* This can best be said as "spon-dil-o" followed by lisps and stutters. The Greek word *olisthesis* means to slide down a slippery path.

Spondylolisthesis is a more severe pars defect, where the vertebra slips forward. This happens when the pars on both sides of the spine fracture and allow the vertebra to move.

There are four grades of spondylolisthesis: Grade zero is no slippage; grade one is 25 percent slippage; grade two, 50 percent; grade three, 75 percent; and grade four 100 percent. With 25 percent slippage, some people will begin to show the bodily configuration of spondylolisthesis; with 33 percent slippage, most will show change; and with 50 percent slippage, all will show it. People with severe spondylolisthesis have flat "heart-shaped" buttocks and a short torso, with a sharp break between the two.

Dr. Jensen treated one elite gymnast with spondylolisthesis who required two screws and a spinal fusion to reconnect her back properly. Although many gymnasts with spondylolisthesis remain in gymnastics, this girl had to leave the sport. However, she went on to become a national class diver.

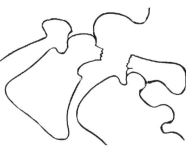

Spondylolisthesis involves a pars break.

The drawing here illustrates Grade one spondylolisthesis. Although the defect may be closed when the gymnast holds the spine in extension (A), separation can occur when the gymnast bends forward.

Causes:

Spondylolisthesis results from the many of the same things that cause stress fractures and spondylolysis. If the above conditions are caught and treated, you are much less likely to have spondylolisthesis happen to you! This condition can also arise in non-athletes, which indicates that some people have a genetic predisposition.

111

Symptoms:

Because spondylolisthesis can happen gradually from a series of stress fractures, you may not be aware that you have it until a crisis. A crisis includes pain, very tight hamstrings, and a peculiar gait. In extreme conditions, a characteristic body deformity develops.

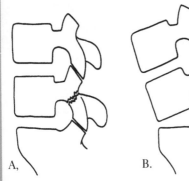

A,   B.

Grade one spondylolisthesis showing slippage as the spine is flexed.

Diagnosis:

Again, x-rays and bone scans are the key diagnostic tools.

Treatment:

One piece of good news is that this condition seldom progresses past the age of 14. The condition can show up as early as five years old, and it is most likely to progress during growth spurts between the ages of nine and 14.

The most common treatment is to stay away from vigorous activity until pain and muscle spasms subside completely, which can take from a few weeks to several months. Use back conditioning exercises and hamstring flexibility exercises, as advised by your doctor. Once the pain goes away and stays away, you can resume all your activities, including competitive gymnastics.

Here are some general guidelines:

■ *Grade one:* If there are no symptoms, you can continue all activities.

■ *Grade two:* You should refrain from sports with high potential of back injury. However, you can participate

112

in other sports, such as swimming and possibly diving. Your doctor should also monitor the slippage with x-rays every six months.

- *Grade three and four:* For people who have more than 50 percent slippage and any symptoms at all, we generally recommend a spinal fusion. We also recommend fusion for people with less slippage but who have continuing back pain and other symptoms, such as hamstring tightness or radiating pain that indicates pressure on the nerve roots.

Vertebral Body Fracture and Scheurmann's Disease

So far, the problems we've talked about have related mostly to the lumbar (lower) spine. Alas, the thoracic spine (the part connected to the rib cage) is not immune to problems.

Sometimes the end plates of the vertebral bodies can fracture, particularly around the front edges. If this isn't allowed to heal properly, it can cause the front edge of the vertebral body to degenerate so that the whole thing becomes wedge-shaped instead of cylindrical. When this happens to several vertebrae in the thoracic spine, you have Scheurmann's disease.

We mentioned kyphosis earlier as forward curvature or humped back. Scheurmann's is an exaggeration of kyphosis, and in early stages it masquerades as big muscular shoulders. What appears to be shoulder and back muscle is, however, the optical illusion caused by a curving spine and the wishful thinking of gymnasts and parents.

In Scheurmann's disease, three or more vertebral bodies of the thoracic spine become wedge-shaped, and the more wedge-shaped they become, the more the spine curves forward.

This condition should not be ignored. Early treatment brings the best results.

Causes:

Repeated small traumas to the vertebra from hyperflexion can cause microscopic vertebral-body fractures. Young people with sway backs that don't curl forward easily may cause these micro-fractures by curling their upper backs more than they should. When the front edges of the vertebral bodies start to degenerate under the stress, the whole vertebral body becomes wedge shaped.

Other causes of Scheurmann's disease are not clearly known. Some of it may be due to a genetic predisposition or simply to an out-of-balance growth spurt.

Symptoms:

The main symptoms are pain and a humped appearance to the back.

Diagnosis:

Normally, x-rays are enough to determine the serious-ness of the condition. Your doctor may also use bone scans.

Treatment:

For mild cases, strengthening exercises and changing workout routines can help balance the spine and remove the source of the condition. For more serious cases, we use braces to immobilize the back and take the pressure off the front of the spine.

Most symptoms disappear in three to four weeks, and you can go back to gymnastic training as long as you have no more symptoms. Bracing may continue for four to six months.

Again, early treatment brings the best results.

Disc Problems

You hear about "slipped discs," but there is no such thing. What happens is that the outside of the disc gets weak and the jelly inside starts to bulge out. Or the disc tears and the jelly leaks out. Bulging or leaking jelly presses on the spinal cord or other nerves and *ow!*

The correct medical term is "herniated" disc, and fortunately it almost never happens to young people.

Symptoms:

Back pain may be relatively minor. Instead, you're more likely to notice a loss of hamstring flexibility or else radiating pain down one or both legs. You may also have trouble flexing your spine (curving forward), and it may be painful to straighten your spine after flexing it.

Diagnosis:

Diagnosis may be difficult. Your doctor will have you make certain moves to determine which cause pain. Since x-rays don't show discs, you may need an MRI scan.

Treatment:

The primary treatment is conservative—rest in a neutral position and avoiding further pain or muscle spasm. That means bed rest, until all pain disappears. In most cases, this is all it takes, but if you return to workouts too soon, you can really mess things up. You don't really want a spinal fusion, do you? No. So follow your doctor's orders. Even if it means staying away from the gym for six to 12 months.

In many cases, braces can allow you to resume activity earlier, depending on the seriousness of the condition.

Overall, disc problems can be something that keeps you away from gymnastics. One study reported that only about 50 percent of patients with disc problems were able to return to full sports activities without pain.[18]

If the disc problem is serious enough to give you bladder and bowel problems or loss of muscle function, you will probably require surgery.

Tumors and Infection

Even though both of these are extremely unlikely, they can't be eliminated. The incidence of bone cancer (osteogenic sarcoma) is low in any age group, but the adolescent and young adult are among the most susceptible.

Discitis (inflammation and infection of the disc) is also unusual but possible, as is infection of the small muscles of the spine. Meningitis is an infection in the spinal canal.

These are possibilities you look for only when all other prospects have played out and back pain remains.

TROUBLESHOOTING: A "DIAGNOSIS" CHART

Here is a quick reference guide when you have a back problem. Please don't think it is the final answer, or that you can use this book instead of checking with your doctor!

*Troubleshooting
your back.*

Symptoms and Diagnosis	Acute pain	Chronic pain	Positive x-ray	Positive MRI or CAT scan	Positive bone scan	Fever	Weight loss, loss of appetite	Positive lab tests
Sprains and strains	✓							
Scoliosis		✓	✓					
Spondylolysis		✓	✓	✓				
Spondylolisthesis		✓	✓	✓				
Vertebral body fracture	✓		✓	✓	✓			
Scheurmann's disease			✓					
Herniated disc		✓		✓				
Tumor		✓		✓		✓	✓	✓
Infections		✓				✓		✓

SUMMARY

Well, it's been a long chapter. Congratulations for sticking with it. The important thing to remember is that most back problems are not serious—but don't ignore them. See a doctor if *any* back pain lasts more than two weeks!

You can help prevent back problems with good conditioning. That means slow, static stretches, plus strengthening work that includes both your back and abdominal muscles. It may or may not be true that the key to a man's heart is his stomach, but it certainly is true that the key to a gymnast's back is her or his stomach.

Be extra careful of your back during growth spurts. Think about it: All your bones are suddenly getting longer and heavier—can your muscles always keep up? No. Muscles need time to adapt to the bigger job they have to do. And *you* need to give them the time.

Finally, if you do get injured, be sure to follow your doctor's orders for complete rehabilitation. No sport, no honor is worth permanently crippling your spine. You live with gymnastics for a few years of your life. You live with your back for the remainder.

[14] McAuley E, Hudash G, Shields K, Albright JP, Garrick J, Requa R, Wallace RK: Injuries in women's gymnastics. *Am J Sports Med* 15:558-565, 1987

[15] Jackson DW, Wiltse LL, Cirincione RJ: Spondylolysis in the female gymnast. *Clin Orthop* 117:68, 1976.

[16] Jackson DW, et al, ibid.

[17] Pettrone FA, Ricciardelli E: Gymnastic injuries: the Virginia experience 1982-83. *Am J Sports Med* 15:59-62, 1987.

[18] Micheli LJ, Hall JF, and Miller ME: Use of the modified Boston brace for back injuries in athletes. *Am J Sports Med* 8:351-356, 1980.

CHAPTER 7

The Knee and Thigh

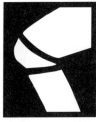

Think about the knee as a hinge, and you'll be about half right. Like a hinge, nearly all the knee's motion is confined to one direction. The knee tolerates only a small amount of rotation and virtually no side-to-side motion, unlike the shoulder and hip, which handle twisting and turning with careless ease.

But the knee differs from a hinge in a big way: The knee has no pin running through the joint to keep it stable. Imagine the system you'd need to keep a door in place if you couldn't use pins in the hinges!

For stability, the knee relies on an intricate system of cartilage and ligaments, tendons and muscles, and even an extra bone—the kneecap or "patella." While we humans have yet to devise an artificial replacement that comes close to being as good as the knee nature makes, the natural version is still a very vulnerable joint. Statistics show that knees are the second leading cause (behind back injuries) for visits to orthopedic surgeons.

As a gymnast, you're most likely to injure your knees in a poor landing or dismount. Just walking up the stairs creates pressures in your knees that are about four times your body weight. And landing from several feet in the air multiplies this force by many times.

THE STRUCTURE OF THE KNEE

Bones and Ligaments

The basic structure of the knee includes four bones and four ligaments. The femur (thigh bone) on the top connects to the tibia (shin bone) and to the fibula (the small leg bone that does not bear weight). The groove in the front of the femur is the "femoral groove," the track that the patella rides in. And the bump on the front of the tibia is the "tibial tuberosity," where the patellar tendon attaches. We'll say more about the patella in a bit.

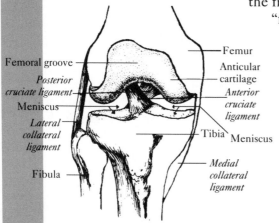

The major bones and ligaments of the knee.

Four primary ligaments hold the bones together: The "medial collateral ligament" on the inside (medial side) of the knee; "the lateral collateral ligament" on the outside (lateral side) of the knee; and two larger ligaments, "the cruciate ligaments" in the center of the knee.

The word "cruciate" originates from the word "cross" or "crucifix," which reflects the fact that the two ligaments cross over each other. The stronger of the two ligaments is the "posterior cruciate ligament" (PCL), which runs from the posterior (back) outside part of the joint towards the front inside. The other and more famous ligament is the "anterior cruciate ligament" (ACL), which runs from the anterior (front) inside part of the joint to the back outside. The PCL almost always

120

remains intact in sports; the ACL is the one that brings people to their knees and their orthopedists.

Cartilage

The drawing also shows the two types of cartilage found in the knee: the "articular cartilage" and the meniscal cartilage or "meniscus."

The articular cartilage covers the end of the femur and the top of the tibia, and it also coats the inside of the patella. This cartilage absorbs shocks and is very slippery, which enables the knee to move easily. Additional lubrication is provided by synovial fluid in the joint.

Damage to the articular cartilage heals slowly. If it gets worn away, you can end up with arthritis.

While the articular cartilage can absorb some shock, most of that job falls to the meniscus.

There are two meniscal cartilages in the knee, each shaped like a crescent c. The outside edge of the crescent is thicker and bears about 70 percent of the weight and shock that the knee is subject to. The meniscus also helps keep the femur and tibia from rubbing one another and wearing out the articular cartilage; people who lose their meniscus due to knee injuries are at a high risk of knee arthritis later in life.

Tendons and Patella

Several tendons attach the muscles to the knee and hold the patella in place.

The patella is nature's answer to the pin in the hinge: It is the fulcrum, the central point of leverage for the knee. When your leg is straight, the patella sits loosely, under no load. As you flex your leg, the patella slides down the femoral groove, and the tendons anchoring it become taut.

In a way, the tendons that attach to the patella act like reins that hold it in place. If the pressure is balanced between the reins (and if there is no knee-joint alignment problem), the patella moves predictably and without problems. If this pressure is thrown off—either by a sudden heavy impact or by a training problem that creates uneven strength in the muscles attached to the various tendons—the patella can become dislocated.

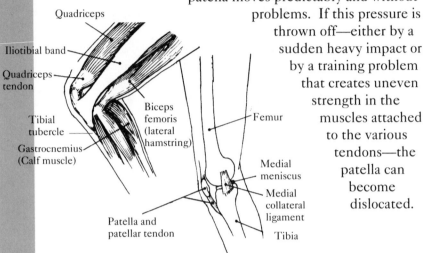

The tendons of the knee, and the kneecap or patella.

COMMON KNEE AND HAMSTRING PROBLEMS

Problems with the knee and hamstring generally fall into four categories: overuse, muscle strains, patellar problems, and acute injuries to ligaments and cartilage. A few miscellaneous problems (like joint mice and Osgood-Schlatter's disease) complete the picture.

In this section, we'll cover the injuries in order by frequency of occurrence. For more information about the general nature of such problems as tendinitis, see the chapter on Body Basics.

Tendinitis

Causes:
Tendinitis generally results from overuse. Too much stress on a poorly conditioned tendon can cause the irritation that leads to inflammation.

The problem can be acute or chronic. For example, you might get acute tendinitis of the patella if you spent several hours doing nothing but landings on a hard surface. If you keep on training the same way and continue to irritate the tendon, the problem may very well become chronic and much more difficult to fix.

Runners typically get tendinitis on the lateral side of their knees, in the iliotibial track, but most gymnasts get tendinitis in the hamstring tendon or in the patellar tendon. Patellar tendinitis is sometimes called "jumper's knee," because it is so common in basketball and volleyball.

Symptoms:
One way to distinguish tendinitis from other knee injuries is that with tendinitis you can continue to use the knee, which makes it possible to continue making the injury worse. It's easy to ignore tendinitis, too, because the stiffness and pain may go away after the first 15 minutes or so of warmup. You don't feel the pain during your workout—but your knee does, and the next day the startup pain will be a little worse. Pay attention and treat the injury before it really settles in and makes your life miserable!

Sometimes tendinitis will cause a grating or sandy feeling over the tendon, which reflects irritation of the tendon where it moves through its sheath. Pain from tendinitis can also radiate along the tendon to the body of the muscle. Severe tendinitis will show some swelling over the area.

Treatment:
Treat tendinitis of the knee as you would any other tendinitis. For an acute injury, apply RICE (that's Rest, Ice,

Compression and Elevation) until the swelling plateaus, then use heat before workouts and ice afterwards. For at least two weeks, arrange your workouts to go light on your knees—avoid hard landings! Also, take aspirin or another anti-inflammatory medicine until the injury heals.

For chronic tendinitis, use heat or contrast therapy and massage. In both cases, acute and chronic, once the injury has healed, you should exercise the muscles attached to the injured tendon to strengthen them and prevent a recurrence.

One other thing—be sure you stretch thoroughly before your workout. That will help prevent tendinitis, and it will also help it heal faster. Stretches must be slow and gradual. No bouncing!

Hamstring Strain

Causes:

As a gymnast, you require incredibly flexible hamstrings to be able to place your body in the positions you do. If the hamstring isn't warmed up properly (slowly and gradually, using controlled stretches), and if you place a sudden load on it, it may tear instead of stretching normally.

Muscles lose elasticity when they get tired, so you're more likely to tear a hamstring if you prolong a workout after your body cries *uncle.*

Hamstring strains are relatively common and can occur almost anywhere in the muscle, from the origin at the ischial tuberosity of the pelvis (the two bones you sit on) to the insertion on the upper tibia.

It's interesting that you can get tendinitis as well as a hamstring strain at or near the ischial tuberosity, which can make gymnastics a pain in the rear, at least temporarily.

Hamstring injuries can be subtle as well as obvious, as one elite gymnast showed. When Dr. Jensen checked her, she could take her right foot all the way over the top of her head, but her left leg missed that by several inches. In a normal

124

examination, you'd think the amount of flexibility in her left hamstring was acceptable, but in comparison with her right hamstring, the left was injured.

Symptoms:

Most hamstring strains happen suddenly, and you'll know it because it'll feel like you've been kicked. Perhaps that's why we hear the term Charley Horse so often. The pain comes from the muscle contracting suddenly in a spasm, its natural defense against excessive stretching.

Treatment:

Use ice immediately to anesthetize the area, and then slowly stretch out the muscle. Massage can be very useful: Sometimes if you maintain heavy pressure at the point of spasm for a few minutes, you can relieve it. If the spasm does not subside, you may need a muscle relaxant. Take aspirin or ibuprofen to prevent inflammation.

Once the acute phase is past, use a neoprene pant or an elastic bandage in a figure-eight wrap to keep the muscle warm, rest the muscle and give it some time to recuperate. Remember, you have some degree of torn tissue in there, and it needs time to grow back together. Fortunately, you're highly unlikely to ever require surgery, even if the muscle is seriously ruptured.

Ligament Sprain

Causes:

Ligament sprains result from abnormal stress on the joint. In short, you've done something wrong. You've missed your dismount, landed badly, tripped or in some way tried to make your knee bend in a direction that nature didn't intend.

The collateral ligaments give way when the knee is forced sideways—football players are especially prone to this when hit. The ACL snaps if you twist the knee too much, or if something tries to bend your leg frontwards instead of backwards.

Symptoms:

Symptoms include pain (from severe to excruciating) and a possibly audible "pop!" The pain may go away for a while, but don't take any chances, because the absence of pain may not mean anything. For example, if you've completely severed a ligament, you may also have severed the pain nerves that would tell you that something is seriously wrong! A feeling of instability in the knee is another sign of ligament damage.

If you hear a loud pop, and your knee swells up almost immediately (indicating blood in the joint), you have a 72 percent chance of having ruptured your ACL.

Even if the signs and symptoms aren't so dramatic, ligament damage is serious and must be examined by a doctor. Put some ice on your knee and take it to one!

Treatment:

Treating a ligament tear depends on how much damage you did to it. Spraining a collateral ligament may require an immobilization splint or cast for three to six weeks. More severe injuries can require surgery.

If possible during recovery, swim a lot. It's a great way to rebuild muscle tone without the strain of gravity.

Meniscus Tear

Causes:

You can tear the meniscus the same way you tear a ligament—sometimes you can really score and injure both at the same time. Any severe twisting, torquing, weight-bearing maneuver with the knee is especially dangerous for the meniscus.

As a gymnast, you should be aware that an MRI scan can show changes in the meniscus due to the pounding your knees take; these changes may look like a tear, but they are not, and they do not require treatment. If your doctor diagnoses a meniscal tear using an MRI, you may want a second opinion.

Symptoms:

How do you tell a meniscus tear from an ACL injury, since the sensation of excruciating pain may be quite similar? Well, you don't, and your doctor does. Having said that, a cartilage tear will often be tender at the joint line between the femur and tibia, while an ACL injury will not.

Also, if the knee locks in one position (it may also release, then lock again), it's a good indicator of a meniscal tear: The loose cartilage is getting in the way of normal motion. If your knee pops, locks or catches in any way, go to your doctor immediately.

Treatment:

Ironically, the most severe injuries heal the quickest. If you tear your meniscus so badly that it cannot be repaired, it can easily be removed by arthroscopic surgery, and you'll be back on the bars feeling fine in three weeks. While this may sound like the ideal solution, it is far from it. Studies have shown that people who have a meniscus removed in their twenties are likely to develop arthritis in the knee by the age of 45 or 50. Nature has a reason for most everything, and we remove "unnecessary" stuff at our peril.

In most cases meniscal tears occur in the inner 70 percent of the cartilage, which you recall carries only 30 percent of the weight. In many cases, it's possible with arthroscopy to remove only the inner part of the meniscus and leave the rest intact. A partial meniscectomy has much the same recovery time-frame as a total removal, and it's a far better solution.

The best solution for the future of the knee and the long-term mobility of the gymnast is to repair the tear in the meniscus, which is possible if the tear is fairly clean. Unfortunately, this solution carries a price in terms of recovery: four months or more. However, when you consider that four months is only 1/240 of your whole life (assuming you live to 80), the option of being an active old lady instead of a crippled old crone is clearly superior.

Chondromalacia patella

Chondromalacia is a mouthful that comes from "chondro" meaning cartilage and "malacia" meaning degeneration. In this case, we're talking about the degeneration of the articular cartilage on the underside of the patella. It's actually a form of localized arthritis.

Causes:
The cause of chondromalacia is improper tracking of the patella in the femoral groove. In a well-designed knee, the patella tracks evenly and exerts equal pressure on all sides. But if the patella tracks unevenly, there's too much pressure in one area, and the articular cartilage there can wear away. There are several reasons for improper tracking:

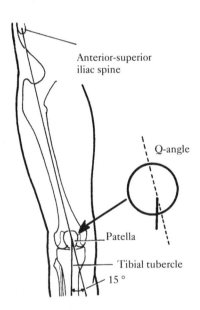

The "Q" angle, showing an angle of 15 degrees

■ The Q-angle is the angle formed by a line drawn down the quadriceps to the knee and a line drawn from the knee down the patella. As you can see from the drawing, if this angle is too large, the patella will naturally be pulled to the outside of the knee. Any angle greater than 20 degrees means increased risk of knee pain and chondromalacia. If you are "knock-kneed," you might want to consider another sport. Girls become more vulnerable to chondromalacia as they mature, because the widening of their hips increases the Q-angle.

- Poor training. If you work out with weights and don't take great care to strengthen all muscles evenly, the uneven strains on the patella can lead to problems.

- Poor metabolism within the articular cartilage. We don't know for sure, but it appears that nature has given some people "Brand X" cartilage, and it simply wears away too easily. This could be another reason to consider a career in a low-impact sport.

Symptoms:

Chondromalacia starts with vague knee pain. Perhaps the patella will grate or crunch when the knee bends. Pain gets worse when you stress the patella by walking downhill, lunging or squatting. Pressing on the patella causes pain, and as the disease gets worse, swelling and tenderness can spread to the knee in general.

Treatment:

There's no guaranteed cure for chondromalacia, since so much of it depends on the way the body is constructed. One thing to do is a balanced exercise program that strengthens the quadriceps, which will reduce the stress on the patella. Bicycling in low gears with the seat up as high as possible is a good form of exercise. Anti-inflammatory medicine may help.

Kneecap Dislocation

Causes:

The same mal-alignment of the patella that causes chondromalacia can also cause the kneecap to dislocate and slip entirely off the front of the knee when there is a lot of stress on kneecap. We have seen this happen when a gymnast lands with his or her feet too far apart.

People with this problem can often push the kneecap out of joint with their hands! While "double-jointed" flexibility is generally good for gymnasts, it's not something you want to see in your kneecap. This problem is frequently inherited.

Symptoms:

This one is pretty obvious. Besides the knee giving way and the severe pain, there are some visual clues that the kneecap is not where it's supposed to be!

Treatment:

If dislocation has not happened more than three times, the treatment is an exercise program designed to strengthen the muscles that hold the patella in place. If the kneecap continues to dislocate, surgery may be able to correct the instability.

Osgood-Schlatter's Disease

If you've been wondering why we labeled the tibial tuberosity in the drawing, here is the answer: The tibial tuberosity is the site for an unusual disease that cures itself.

The tibial tuberosity, besides being the place where the patellar tendon attaches, is also a growth plate (an apophysis). It is almost a separate piece of bone separated from the tibia by a fissure line where new growth takes place.

Bone growing out from the fissure line around the tibial tuberosity adds to the circumference of the tibia, but this growing bone also makes the tibial tuberosity a weak area. Irritation can develop here, leading to inflammation called tibial tuberculitis or Osgood-Schlatter's disease. Note that this is *not* tibial tuberculosis!

In an extreme form, the tibial tuberosity can actually break off. We showed an x-ray of this in the chapter on Body Basics.

Causes:

The cause of Osgood-Schlatter's disease is not really known. It may be that the quadriceps muscle is too weak, allowing too much force to be transmitted to the attachment of the quad at the tibial tuberosity.

Symptoms:

This condition produces pain in front of the knee, right at the "bump." The pain gets worse with strenuous activity, like running and gymnastics.

Treatment:

At about the age of 14 in girls and 16 in boys, the growth line fuses, the bone becomes one solid piece, and the disease cures itself. While you wait for age, work to strengthen your quadriceps.

Joint Mouse

A *joint mouse* is one of those colorful terms in medicine that keep us from succumbing to too much Latin. A stuffier name is a "loose body." Joint mice live within the knee. They can start out small and harmless and end up a real nuisance, not by multiplying but by growing larger.

Causes:

If you injure your knee, you may inadvertently chip off a bit of cartilage that's left to float around. Initially there are very few symptoms—nothing more than the occasional snap or crackle. However, as the little mouse floats around in the synovial fluid, it grows much like a pearl inside an oyster, and often becomes big enough to cause problems.

Symptoms:

Symptoms are much like a torn knee cartilage, including snapping, popping, swelling, pain and giving way in the knee. The best way to tell a joint mouse from torn cartilage is x-ray or MRI.

Treatment:

The joint mouse should be trapped and removed. Normally, this is a simple arthroscopic procedure with a short three-week recovery time.

Synovitis

Causes:

The synovium is the lining of the knee joint, and like other tissues of the body it can become irritated and inflamed. The most common causes of synovitis are torn cartilage, joint mice or chondromalacia.

When the synovium gets irritated, it makes more synovial fluid and the joint swells up. Sometimes this condition is called "water on the knee." Synovitis can also occur as an overuse injury.

Symptoms:

Synovitis can cause mild discomfort to severe pain that completely prevents putting weight on the knee. There is also generalized swelling.

Treatment:

If staying off the knee for a while doesn't help, see your doctor to determine the cause. You may require surgery to remove a joint mouse.

Knee Braces

Obviously, knee braces aren't a "common knee and hamstring problem," but sometimes they can help solve a problem. They come in several flavors:

Wraps

The elastic wrap alone offers no real structural support, but it does provide warmth for healing, plus some psychological benefit. Some people wear a wrap instead of seeing their doctor—but a brace is no substitute for medical care!

Preventive braces

The two most common preventive braces are the McDavid Knee Guard and the Anderson Knee Stabler, both of which limit side-to-side motion and use stays and hinges to prevent twisting.

Basketball and football players often use these braces, but the scientific evidence about their value is mixed. Some coaches are convinced that knee braces prevent injuries; while some studies suggest braces actually increase injuries.

Using a brace if you don't have a problem could provide a false sense of security, because no brace can substitute for strength and balance.

Functional and custom braces

Functional braces are prescribed by a physician and may be quite complex and expensive. These braces use titanium and other exotic alloys to provide relatively light-weight protection for gymnasts as they train in the months following surgery (an ACL repair, for example). Some physicians prescribe these braces for gymnasts whose ligaments are naturally lax; however, we believe that if you require this kind of brace to avoid injury you should consider choosing another sport.

Postoperative braces

Postoperative braces are used immediately after surgery to restrict the knee's range of motion but allow enough movement to prevent muscle atrophy. Most braces are adjustable so that the range of motion can be increased as healing progresses.

TROUBLESHOOTING: A "DIAGNOSIS" CHART

Here is a quick reference guide when you have a knee problem. Please don't think it is the final answer, or that you can use this book instead of checking with your doctor!

*Troubleshooting
your knees.*

Symptoms and Diagnosis	Acute pain	Chronic pain recurrent	Acute swelling	Late swelling (>24 hrs)	Pop!	Locking	Grinding	Giving way
Tendinitis	✔	✔						
Hamstring strain	✔							
Ligament sprain	✔		✔					✔
Meniscus tear		✔	✔	✔	✔	✔	✔	✔
Chondromalacia patella		✔		✔		✔	✔	
Kneecap dislocation	✔		✔		✔			✔
Osgood-Schlatter's		✔		✔				
Joint mouse		✔		✔		✔		
Synovitis		✔		✔				

135

SUMMARY

In this chapter, we've talked about how the knee works and some of the things that can go wrong. Most knee injuries heal quickly *if you take care of them*. Yes, we know that as a young person you know you are both immortal and indestructible, but . . .

The message is, If anything odd about your knees persists more than a day or two, see your doctor! There is life after gymnastics, and it's not nearly as much fun if you can't use your knees.

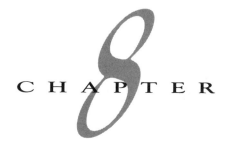

C H A P T E R

The Shoulder, Elbow and Wrist

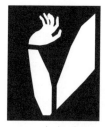

You gymnasts use arms the way other people use legs. And you swing from them enough to put a monkey to shame. Not surprising then, that orthopedists see so many injuries to shoulders, elbows and wrists.

In this chapter, we'll cover anatomy and the most common injuries. We'll also have some tips to prevent injury.

THE SHOULDER

The way the arm connects with the rest of the body is almost spooky. While the leg uses tough ligaments at every joint, the shoulder gets by with a little help from its muscles. The shoulder joint has the greatest range of motion and the least stability of any joint in the body.

The upper arm (the *humerus*) fits rather loosely into the shoulder blade (*scapula*). Like the hip, the shoulder is a ball-and-socket joint, but there the similarity ends. It's very unusual for people to dislocate a hip, but shoulder dislocations are unfortunately not difficult to achieve.

The shoulder joint is less stable than the hip for three reasons:

■ The socket in the scapula is shallow compared to the socket in the pelvis.

- There are fewer and smaller ligaments tying the humerus to the scapula compared to those that tie the femur to the pelvis.

- The scapula has no direct connections to the spine, while the pelvis is actually part of the spine.

Structure of the Shoulder

Bones, ligaments and bursae

The drawing shows the bones of the shoulder joint, viewed from the front. The *acromion* (you can only see its front tip in this drawing) is the projection of a spiny ridge that runs along the back of the scapula. Reach behind your back and feel the acromion with your hand, starting at the tip of your shoulder and slanting downward toward your spine.

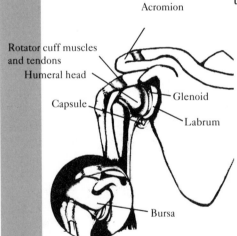

Acromion

Rotator cuff muscles and tendons

Humeral head

Capsule

Glenoid

Labrum

Bursa

Structure of the shoulder joint.

The socket (called the *glenoid*) nestles right below the acromion. Around the edge of the socket sits the *labrum* (this comes from the Latin word for "lip"), which is cartilage much like the meniscus in the knee. The labrum helps make the socket a little deeper, so the joint is a bit more stable. The bony finger that juts out of the scapula is the *coracoid process*. Coracoid comes from the Greek word *korakaeides* meaning "like a raven"—a reference to the bird-beak shape. (And have you noticed that things that stick out of bones are always called "processes"?)

138

The drawing does not show the ligaments that connect the arm to the shoulder blade. In the armpit, ligaments connect the humerus to the scapula. On top, ligaments run from the humerus to the coracoid process, and from the coracoid process to the acromion and the clavicle.

Confused yet? Don't worry about these ligaments, because the real work of holding the arm in place falls to the rotator cuff muscles.

Before we get to the rotator cuff muscles, we want to mention one other important feature of the shoulder: the *bursae*. The bursa shown in the illustration sits like a cap on the head of the humerus, in the space between the humerus and the underside of the acromion. This bursa cushions the joint, and you'll hear more about it when we talk about injuries.

The rotator cuff

There are three rotator cuff muscles on the back side of the scapula, so named because they rotate the arm to the outside. The *supraspinatus* ("above the spine") is at the top above the acromion, the *infraspinatus* ("below the spine") is in the middle, and the *teres minor* is at the bottom. Sometimes we call these the SIT muscles, from the first letter of each name.

Supraspinatus
Deltoid
Infraspinatus
Teres minor

The rotator cuff muscles, posterior view.

On the front side of the scapula the subscapularis muscle rotates the arm inward.

You can't feel any of these muscles through the skin, because they all lie underneath other muscles; however, they're

139

quite important. The SIT muscles stabilize the ball-and-socket joint and they help raise your arm, as well as rotate it.

You're probably familiar with the deltoid—it's the big muscle that runs around the outside of the shoulder, and it's right there to see in the mirror. You may think the deltoid is the most important muscle in raising your arm (and it is important), but you would never get started without the SITs.

One important thing to note about the rotator cuff muscles is that the tendons that connect them to the humerus have a tight squeeze. These tendons must scrunch in between the acromion and the humeral head, underneath the bursa. This crowded space can cause problems, one of which is a "rotator cuff tear," which we'll talk more about later.

We could probably spend another ten pages describing all the muscles of the shoulder. With back and front, top, underside, and multiple layers, you have what can only be described as a plethora.

Why so many? Because your shoulder girdle can slide around in many directions, it takes bunches of muscles to control. The knee moves in two directions, so it takes only two sets of muscles (quadriceps and hamstrings).

Here's another feature special to the shoulder: Most of the muscles work most of the time! In the knee, the quadriceps contracts while the hamstrings relax, and vice versa. But getting the exact arm movement you want requires balanced contractions of many muscles working together. Muscle balance is the big word for the shoulder.

Impingement Problems

Nature designed the arm to spend most of its time hanging from your shoulder, close to your side. Any sport that requires continual overhead arm action (like tennis serves, baseball pitching, gymnastics, etc.) puts stress on the joint.

When you raise your arm out to the side and over your head, you may notice that it's easier if your palms are up instead of down. When you turn your palms up, this external rotation (the thumb rotates outward) opens up a little more space for the humerus to rotate upwards. When you internally rotate your arm (turn your thumb down—for example in a tennis serve or overhead pitch) you squeeze the space between the acromion and the humeral head. This means you also squeeze the rotator cuff tendons (particularly the supraspinatus) and the bursa. If you don't have quite enough room in this area, or if you abuse your shoulder with too much overhead motion and not enough time to repair damage, you can irritate these tissues.

Now we have the possibility of a nasty cycle setting in: Continual irritation of the rotator cuff tendons and bursa causes swelling and scarring. The thickened tissue impinges even more and gets further irritated.

Impingement is an overuse problem: The body's repair mechanisms can't keep up with the damage inflicted. Eventually, the rotator cuff can tear. Then you have serious discomfort.

Causes:

In gymnastics, the major cause of impingement problems is the amount of time spent your arms raised over your head. Your shoulders also experience a considerable jolt every time you vault or flip.

Another possible cause is ligament laxity. Gymnasts with the most flexible ligaments may have the most shoulder problems because the shoulder ligaments are not holding the humeral head tightly in the glenoid. Seriously lax ligaments can lead to instability problems and dislocations, which we'll talk about in a bit.

Symptoms:

If your shoulder swells up or hurts for more than a week, or if you have real trouble raising your arm, see a doctor.

Treatment:

Simple muscle strains should get well within a week, using RICE initially, followed by alternating heat and cold treatments and gentle exercise. Pain that lasts longer could be serious and should be seen and diagnosed by a doctor.

Treatment includes anti-inflammatory medication, heat and cold treatment, ultrasound and microelectric nerve stimulation. One important treatment (when you catch impingement problems at an early stage) is strengthening exercises using rubber cords. The strengthening program should be guided by a sports medicine specialist or trainer, because if you strengthen one muscle too much, you can throw off the muscle balance system and lose your flexibility. It's also important not to work too hard on a strengthening program, or you can actually worsen the problem.

Sometimes surgery will be required to clear a space and prevent impingement. Nowadays, surgery is much more sophisticated and less debilitating than it was only a few years ago. Linda had an open-shoulder operation for a torn rotator cuff in the mid-eighties (before she met Dr. Jensen) and was in the hospital several days on morphine. At the time, she wished she'd just told them to amputate.

Dr. Jensen says these operations are much easier nowadays because surgery can be done arthroscopically or semi-arthroscopically. He does shoulder surgery as an outpatient procedure, with a small incision and minimal damage to surrounding tissue.

Surgical options for opening space include:

■ Shaving off torn and irritated rotator cuff and sewing together tears.

■ Removing a thickened and damaged bursa. (If it is severely damaged, it isn't doing any good anyway.)

■ Trimming the underside of the acromion bone.

142

Stay away from steroid injections into the rotator cuff. They can soften and weaken the cuff and make it even more likely to tear. Linda's tear followed several "Dr. Brand X" cortisone injections that temporarily helped symptoms but worsened the damage.

Instability and Subluxation

While shoulders can dislocate and come out of the socket altogether, it's much more common to see partial dislocation, which is also called *subluxation*. This is a shoulder instability problem.

The arm can subluxate in three directions: forwards, backwards or downwards. It can't move upwards, because the acromion is in the way. Forward subluxation is by far the most common.

Causes:

If you force your shoulder beyond its range of motion, the ball can pop part-way out of the socket. The joint may not dislocate completely, but the tissues that hold it together can become damaged and loose. Capsular ligaments can tear, and the labrum (the lip of cartilage around the edge of the glenoid) can pull loose from the scapula.

Instability can also result from inborn ligament laxity.

Symptoms:

The main symptom is the "dead arm" syndrome. Your arm goes numb and feels like it's temporarily paralyzed. It "goes out" on you—for a few moments it just doesn't work. There will probably be some pain, but nothing compared to what you feel if the shoulder goes all the way out and dislocates.

Subluxation generally doesn't show up on x-rays.

143

Treatment:

Before you let anyone talk you into surgery, try exercises to strengthen the muscles that stabilize the shoulder. This is the most common cure for this problem and can be very successful.

If the shoulder continues to subluxate, you may require either arthroscopic or open surgery. The orthopedic surgeon can tighten and stabilize the joint by reattaching the capsular ligaments and removing or repairing a torn labrum. If the subluxation is serious enough to warrant surgery, returning to gymnastics will be difficult.

Dislocation

Dislocation means that the humeral head comes so far out of the glenoid that it can't snap back in without professional medical intervention. Shoulders can dislocate forwards (most common), backwards or downwards.

Causes:

The most likely cause of shoulder dislocation is a sudden blow or twisting force on the arm. Ligament laxity and shoulder instability may predispose you to shoulder dislocation.

Symptoms:

Dr. Jensen guarantees you will know if your shoulder dislocates!

Treatment:

Don't move, and have someone call an ambulance. Shoulders should be reduced (that means returned to their sockets) by doctors who know what they're doing.

Once the shoulder is back in place, you should follow a careful guided program of strengthening exercises. Shoulders that dislocate more than two to three times may require surgical stabilization.

Labrum Injuries

Causes:

We mentioned that the labrum is cartilage around the glenoid that helps make the socket a little deeper. A dislocation or an unstable joint can tear the labrum, which can cause painful popping and catching when you move your upper arm. The situation is quite similar to damaging the meniscal cartilage in the knee.

Symptoms:

Popping and cracking in the shoulder joint point to a labrum tear. Pain is another symptom. Because subluxation and dislocation can both injure the labrum, be alert for labrum symptoms if these occur.

Treatment:

Like meniscal repair, this repair requires surgery. The orthopedic surgeon will use arthroscopic or open surgery to sew the labrum back together or remove it if the damage is too great.

Recovery generally takes from four to six months, and returning to gymnastics will be difficult.

THE ELBOW

While tennis players have made the elbow famous, gymnasts also know it well. The main problem we see in elbows is tendinitis. Elbow fractures, while less frequent, are serious injuries and can be difficult to repair and recover from.

Clavicle
Acromion
Humerus
Olecranon
Lateral epicondyle
Medial epicondyle
Capitellum
Trochlea
Radius
Ulna
Radial styloid
Ulnar styloid
Carpal bones
Metacarpals
Scaphoid navicular
Phalanges

Bones of the arm, posterior view.

145

As you'll see, there are some things you can do to keep from injuring your elbows.

Structure of the Elbow

The drawing on page 145 shows the entire arm, as viewed from the back. Here you get a better picture of the acromion on the back of the shoulder blade, along with the elbow and wrist.

The long pointy bone on the back of your elbow is the ulna, which starts large next to the humerus and is smaller by the time it reaches your wrist. If you stand with your arm down and your thumb out, the ulna is the lower arm bone closest to your body. The elbow point itself is called the *olecranon*, from the Greek words *olene* (meaning ulna!) and *kranion* (meaning head). This is where the word cranium comes from.

A second bone stretches from the humerus to the thumb: the radius. One way to remember which bone is which, is to think of your *thumb* making circles (fingers can't do this), and then think of the *radius* of a circle.

When you bend your arm, the radius and ulna each slide around the end of the humerus on tracks of their own. The radius slides around the *capitellum*, and the ulna slides around the *trochlea*. These don't show in the drawing, since they're on the front side of the elbow (after all, your arm bends forward, not backward). What does show in the drawing are the *condyles* that stick out to the side of the capitellum and trochlea. Condyles, as you remember, are the rounded bumps on the ends of bones where ligaments and tendons attach. (Comic-strip dogs always bury bones with big condyles.)

There's one elbow bone that's really a nerve: the "funny bone." The ulnar nerve to your hand runs very close to the surface as it passes along the back of your elbow, just to the inside of the ulna. If you whack your elbow just right (or just wrong), you hit the ulnar nerve, and it makes your fourth and fifth fingers tingle.

146

The elbow moves in only two directions and is well stocked with heavy-duty ligaments (medial collateral ligaments on the inside and lateral collateral ligaments on the outside) to make sure that it doesn't move any other way. The biceps muscle on the front side of the humerus flexes the elbow, and the triceps muscle on the back side of the humerus extends it.

Muscles that move your hand and wrist hook up to the elbow at *epicondyles*. (Condyles, epicondyles. . .what is this? Condyles are bumps and epicondyles are bumps on bumps. Perhaps it's like saying the "epicenter" of an earthquake instead of just saying the "center," which would make just as much sense. Anyway, at the elbow, they're called epicondyles.) The muscles that flex your wrist and fingers inward attach to the inside or medial epicondyle. The muscles that extend your wrist and fingers outward attach to the outside or lateral epicondyle.

We'll be that by now you've figured out that medial always means toward the center line of your body, while lateral means away from the center line. Now let's stop a minute and explain flexion and extension. They are confusing enough in the wrist, but wait until you get to the ankle and foot! Consider this a primer.

Wrist extension is when the fingernail side of your hand moves towards the hairy side of your arm: the position your hands are in when you do a handstand. Doctors would say that the dorsum of the wrist comes toward the dorsum of the forearm. Dorsum is medical lingo for "back," like the dorsal fin of a fish is the fin on its back.

Flexion is when the palm of your hand goes toward the forearm.

When your wrist is straight out from the arm in one continuous line, it is neither flexed nor extended, at least in medical terms!

This is all different in the foot. Stay tuned.

Strains and Sprains

Causes:

Strains and sprains can happen in the muscles and ligaments of the arm, just as they can in the rest of the body.

Muscle strains normally are no worse than first or second degree, and they commonly arise from hyperextension. If you fall on an outstretched arm in such a way that it tries to bend your elbow the wrong way, the biceps may be strained as it resists the move.

The same type of fall can also strain the ligaments of the elbow, particularly if there is any sideways force against the joint.

Symptoms:

Strains cause local pain at the point of the muscle damage. If you sprain your elbow, you may feel diffuse pain above the elbow, and you may be unable to grasp an object in that hand because of the pain. If you start poking around with your other hand, you'll find that the source of the pain is the medial collateral ligament on the inside of the elbow, right at the joint. The symptoms are similar to medial epicondylitis (tendinitis— see next page), except that a sprain is an acute injury that happens all at once, while tendinitis is an overuse injury that grows slowly worse over time.

It is possible, although highly unlikely, to completely tear a muscle or a ligament. Only a doctor can diagnose this. Ligament tears may require surgery to correct.

Treatment:

For mild or moderate (first-or second-degree) strains and sprains, treat with RICE. Strains should get better within three weeks, while sprains may take up to six weeks.

Tendinitis

Why did we spend so much time talking about epicondyles earlier? Because the official name of this problem is not really tennis elbow or tendinitis but *epicondylitis.* Regardless of the name, it is the inflammatory response that you should know well by this point in the book.

Causes:

"Tendinitis" can happen on either the medial or lateral epicondyle. The most famous form happens on the lateral side or outside and is the classic "tennis elbow." In tennis, lateral epicondylitis comes from poor backhand form—slapping at the ball by extending your wrist instead of moving your whole arm. You can also get tennis elbow on the medial epicondyle, usually through bad serves. (Again, too much wrist action.) While this book isn't about tennis, we want to give you some idea of the motions that cause tendinitis in the elbow.

The most common form of elbow tendinitis in gymnasts is the medial variety. You get it because of all high-stress flexion you do with your hands and wrists.

Symptoms:

Tendinitis produces local pain, either on the inside or outside of your elbow. The pain can also radiate down into the muscles of the forearm.

Treatment:

For acute tendinitis, use ice and friction massage to help heal inflamed tendons and bursae. Ice constricts surface blood vessels (cutting blood flow), and friction dilates them (promoting blood flow). So why use both? Alternating from one to the other stimulates overall circulation, which helps remove waste products and bring in the raw materials needed for healing.

The easiest way to use ice is to freeze water in paper cups or frozen juice cans. Don't use chemical ice—it can be too

149

cold! Rub the ice around the sore area until it gets numb, about three to four minutes. Then switch to friction massage, rubbing back and forth over the sore spot. Start lightly and gradually increase pressure, until it's quite firm. When feeling returns, use the ice again. End the process with ice to still the inflammation. The whole process takes 15 to 20 minutes, and you should do it two to three times a day.

Once you are free of pain for a few days, start rehabilitation exercises. Do them daily, and apply ice for 20 minutes when you finish. Start by stretching your wrist, using the other hand to bend the hand connected to the wounded elbow first one way then the other. You can do this palm up or palm down, and with your arm bent or straight. Experiment to find the position that seems to stretch the injured area.

Strengthen the muscles by doing wrist curls and reverse curls (up fast, down slow) with a weight that allows 20 to 30 repetitions. Do two sets of each. You can also squeeze a nerf ball or something similar, but keep it to 20 repetitions.

Occasionally, doctors use steroids to halt the inflammatory reaction so the injury can heal. If you get a steroid injection (e.g. Cortisone®), you should really take it easy on that arm for at least one week, so that any tissue damaged by the shot itself can heal.

A new electrical technique called *iontophoresis* can drive cortisone through the skin into the affected tissue. This avoids the pain and inconvenience of a shot altogether.

To help protect your arm during rehabilitation and to help prevent future damage, you may want to use an elbow brace. Braces come in many varieties, from simple below-the-elbow Velcro® straps to more complex above- and below-the-joint contraptions.

Elbow tendinitis can take six to 12 months to heal. If it lasts longer than this, it may require surgery. The important thing is to catch it early. Don't ignore elbow pain!

Dislocation

Causes:

Elbow dislocation is a severe traumatic injury caused by a fall on a straight arm or a sudden violent blow to the elbow.

Symptoms:

You will know if this happens. The pain is immediate and severe, and you can't use your arm, which has the wrong shape. Immobilize the joint and call an ambulance. You will probably require anesthetic to stand having your elbow put back together again, which should only be done by a doctor. Since dislocations frequently come along with broken bones and since young gymnasts may pull off a growth plate, x-rays are mandatory.

Treatment:

If the bones of the elbow have dislocated very far, it may not be possible to snap them back together without surgery.

Even if the doctor is able to reduce the dislocation (put it back together) without surgery, it will still take many months of physical therapy to recover full function. The elbow will probably be splinted until the pain subsides. Dr. Jensen starts dislocation patients on careful, guided range-of-motion exercises as soon as the pain allows it, to avoid muscular atrophy.

It may take four to six months to return to full gymnastics workouts, although some motivate gymnasts make it much sooner than that.

The prognosis for a full recovery from an elbow dislocation is better than for a shoulder dislocation. At least one gymnast has gone from a dislocated elbow to medal performance at the Olympics.

Fractures

Elbow fractures can be really nasty, because a key nerve and an important artery to the hand run very close to the joint.

The worst kind is a supracondylar fracture, where the humerus breaks just above the condyles. These usually require surgery and lengthy rehabilitation.

Elbow fractures can cause lingering stiffness, limitation of motion, growth disturbances and problems with nerves and blood vessels.

The most common cause of elbow fracture, particularly the supracondylar fracture, is a fall on an outstretched arm. By now, you'll have noticed that many unpleasant things can happen as a result of falling on an outstretched arm. You can also break your wrist. The best advice is not to do it. Curl up and relax into a fall. Babies do it because they don't know any better, and good skiers do it because they're tired of getting beaten up and broken.

Supracondylar fractures:

This very serious fracture is a break in the humerus, right above the elbow. It produces severe pain and deformity. Don't move the joint, or you can worsen damage to nerves and blood vessels. *Don't* put any kind of compressive dressing on the break or it can further squash nerves and blood vessels that may already be caught between the ends of the broken bones. If your hand feels cold, stiff or numb, these are important warning signals. In any case, call an ambulance immediately.

Unless this is a hairline fracture and the bone hasn't moved out of place, you will almost certainly require surgery.

Olecranon fractures:

This is where the point of the elbow breaks off, usually as a result of a direct blow. Because the triceps muscle attaches here and keeps pulling the olecranon away from the rest of the humerus, repair of this break usually requires surgery.

Radial head fractures:

The head of the radius can fracture, and if the bone isn't displaced, the break should heal easily with a short period of splinting, followed by guided exercise.

Epicondylar fractures:

The epicondyles are growth plates, and as such have a somewhat weakened connection to the main part of the bone. Surgery may be required to reattach an epicondyle that has broken loose, depending on exactly how loose the epicondyle is.

Osteochondritis desiccans

This is an unusual condition with no clear cause. From the word 'desiccans' you get the idea that something is drying out. Most typically, *osteochondritis desiccans* strikes the *capitellum* (the track in the humerus where the radius rides), which gradually degrades and crumbles.

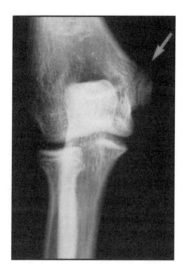

Growth plate on the medial epicondyle of the elbow. The x-ray on the left shows a partially fused growth plate (at the arrow). The line indicates the part of the plate that is still open. The x-ray below shows a growth plate that has been pulled off by the muscles. This gymnast went on to the Olympics.

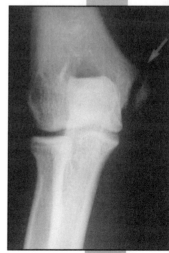

Symptoms and diagnosis:

Any chronic pain on the outside of your elbow that doesn't respond to traditional tendinitis treatments should be reason enough to see a doctor. Your doctor may use x-rays, bone scans, MRI, CAT scans or arthroscopy to make this diagnosis.

Treatment:

Treatment of this condition includes exercise, bracing and continual attention. It may

153

or may not heal. Dr. Jensen has worked with many gymnasts who have this condition: Some stay in the sport, and others are not able to.

THE WRIST

Structure of the Wrist

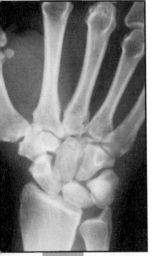

X-ray of an adult wrist. All growth plates are closed in this adult. This x-ray gives a clear view of the carpal bones.

The far ends of the ulna and radius make up the base for the wrist joint. The ulnar styloid marks the end of the ulna—it's the bump on the outside of your wrist. On the other side of your wrist the radial styloid is a less obvious bump.

Eight carpal bones comprise the wrist itself. The word "carpal" probably comes from the Latin word *carpus*, meaning wrist, although it's more interesting to think that it comes from the low Latin word *carp*, a type of fish. All these little bones together might remind you of a school of goldfish.

One of the carpal bones you'll hear more about is the *scaphoid navicular*, near the thumb. Scaphoid comes from the Greek work *skaphe*, meaning a boat, and navicular comes from the Latin word *navicularis*, meaning "pertaining to a small ship or boat." (Our word "navigation" comes from the same root.) Not taking any chances with what this bone looks like!

An amazingly complex system of ligaments and joint capsules interconnects the carpal bones and ties them to the radius and ulna (on the arm side) and to the metacarpals (on the finger side).

You have five metacarpals, one for each of your five fingers. The metacarpals make up the palms of your hands. The finger bones are called *phalanges*.

Most of the muscles for the fingers are in the forearm—to prove it, grip your arm just below the elbow and wiggle your fingers. Feel all those muscles contract? If the finger muscles were actually in the fingers, your fingers would be too fat to move! So you have a marvelous system of tendons that connects finger joints to the strong and bulky muscles in the forearm.

The wrist and hand are the most versatile and functional contraption anywhere in the animal kingdom. And the opposable thumb is a real stroke of genius.

Tendinitis

Causes:

Tendinitis in the wrist results from overuse—too much stress without enough time to recover. It occurs most frequently on the hairy side of the lower arm a few inches above the wrist. It typically lasts about two to three weeks.

Symptoms:

Pain, swelling and tenderness.

Treatment:

Treat it with RICE, and when the pain goes away, strengthen the wrist with wrist curls. You can use the same ice and friction message and the same rehabilitation exercises we described earlier for elbow tendinitis, since the same muscles are involved.

Sprains and Dislocations

You can sprain ligaments in your wrist, but fortunately, it's almost impossible to dislocate the wrist. Since most of the muscles for the hand are in the forearm, wrist strains seldom occur.

A simple sprain should heal in a week or two. If it does not, something else may be wrong. Regardless, it's wise to see your doctor.

Treatment includes RICE and strengthening exercises, much as we described for tendinitis.

Scaphoid Navicular Fracture

The scaphoid navicular is one of the carpal bones, and the most susceptible to fracture. This type of fracture is very difficult to heal and may take months, requiring close attention by your physician.

Causes:

Again, a fall on an outstretched arm can do it. Scaphoid fractures can also arise gradually from overuse, as do stress fractures.

Diagnosis:

These fractures may be difficult to spot on an x-ray; a bone scan will show a "hot spot" if a fracture exists. Your doctor might also use an MRI scan to diagnose this type of fracture.

Treatment:

If the fracture is severe, you might be in a cast for months. For less extreme cases, bracing and taping should be sufficient. There are a number of new wrist braces available, which seem to be quite helpful.

In some cases, you may require surgery to set the bones after a displaced fracture (a fracture where one part of the bone has moved away from the other part).

In all cases, it is important to maintain your overall exercise program and also do exercises to strengthen the wrist.

Radius and Ulna Fractures

The wrist can break at the end of the radius, frequently breaking the tip of the ulna as well. If both bones break, it's called a Colles' fracture.

Again, a growth plate can be the culprit: The wrist can fracture at the epiphyseal growth plate of the radius, where the radius meets the carpal bones. It is important to diagnose and treat this type of fracture, or the plate may close prematurely. If that happens, the radius quits growing while the ulna grows on, which throws the wrist out of balance and even creates deformities—the hand doesn't point in the same direction as the arm! The moral is: Don't ignore wrist pain.

Cause:

We realize that this is getting boring, but a fall on an outstretched arm is a common cause of these fractures. Overuse can cause stress fractures.

Symptoms:

If you fall and break both radius and ulna, you'll know it because your wrist and arm will not look right and the pain will be severe.

Lesser breaks will not hurt as much, but they should not be ignored. Stress fractures are particularly dangerous, in that they creep up on you and can be neglected long past the point where you should have seen your doctor.

Any pain in your wrist should take you to the doctor.

Diagnosis:

An x-ray will show a clean break, while a bone scan may be required to diagnose stress fractures. The sample bone scan in the Body Basics chapter shows the "hot spot" generated by a stress fracture in the left radius at the growth plate.

Treatment:

You may be in a cast for a few weeks; if it's only a stress fracture, you may only be splinted or braced. Treatment is very similar to that for scaphoid navicular fractures. You can continue workouts, but you must avoid stress on the wrist (like vaulting) until the fracture heals.

TFCC Injuries

The knee joint has the meniscus; the shoulder joint has the labrum; and the wrist has the *triangular fibrocartilaginous complex* (called the TFCC for obvious reasons). The TFCC is cartilage material like the meniscus and labrum, and it sits between the ulna and the carpals. Like the meniscus and labrum, the TFCC cushions the joint and helps keep it stable.

Causes:
A sudden twisting injury to the wrist can tear this cartilage.

Symptoms:
Point tenderness just below the ulnar styloid, plus pain when moving the wrist.

Diagnosis:
This will not show up on an x-ray and requires an arthrogram or MRI.

Treatment:
Treatment may include a splint or cast, and in some cases may even require surgery. Recovery time is quite variable.

TROUBLESHOOTING: A "DIAGNOSIS" CHART

Here is a quick reference guide about shoulders, elbows and wrists. Please don't rely on this chart when you should see your doctor!

Troubleshooting your shoulder, elbow and wrist.

Symptoms & Diagnosis	Acute pain	Chronic or reoccurring pain	Acute (immediate) swelling	Late swelling	Positive X-ray	Positive bone scan	Positive MRI
SHOULDER:							
Impingement	✓	✓					✓
Dislocation			✓		✓		✓
Labrum injury		✓					
Instability		✓					
ELBOW:							
Strains	✓✓						
Sprains	✓✓						
Tendinitis		✓					
Dislocation			✓	✓	✓		
Fracture			✓	✓	✓		
Osteochondritis desiccans		✓		✓	✓	✓	✓
WRIST:							
Tendinitis		✓					
Sprains	✓		✓				
Scaphoid fracture	✓			✓	✓	✓	
Radius/ulna fractures	✓		✓	✓	✓		
TFCC injuries	✓	✓					✓

SUMMARY

How to summarize so much in a paragraph or two?
Perhaps in all this there are three main points:

■ Don't ignore pain in your shoulder, elbow or arm. Any
   injury will heal faster if it receives the right treatment as
   soon as possible. This is especially true of tendinitis!
   Listen to your body and get help when it tells you to.
   Most of the time, treatment will not keep you away from
   the sport for long, if at all.

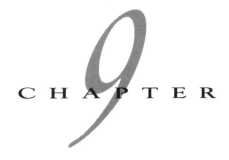

The Leg, Ankle and Foot

Sit on the floor with your legs straight out in front of you. Pull your foot up and move it from side to side. Now push your foot down and move it again. Suddenly it goes farther—all because of a cunning design feature of the *talus bone*.

The leg, ankle and foot come with a number of cunning features designed to take the terrific pounding that comes with having all your weight on two legs. Your legs and ankles also give you remarkable freedom in the ways you can move.

In this chapter, we'll cover basic anatomy, injuries most common to gymnasts, plus preventive and rehabilitative exercises.

BASIC ANATOMY

The leg, ankle and foot really function as one unit, but we'll separate them for discussion. Before we start, let's clear up some confusion we warned you about in the Shoulder, Elbow and Wrist chapter.

Confusing Medical Directions—or,
How Does That Thing Bend?

Whether various parts of your foot flex or extend depends as much on the part you're talking about as it does on the direction of movement. Here goes:

■ *Dorsal flexion* means flexing the dorsal or top surface of the foot by pulling the foot upward.

■ *Plantar flexion* means flexing the bottom (plantar) surface of your foot by pushing it down, as though you were pressing on the accelerator in a car.

■ *Toe extension* means that you are pulling your toes back towards you.

■ *Toe flexion* means that you are curling your toes under your foot.

■ *Pronation* means that your foot leans to the inside.

■ *Supination* means that you have a very high arch and your foot leans to the outside.

■ *Eversion* refers to the ankle and means that it bends outward. Generally, when the ankle everts, the foot pronates.

■ *Inversion* also refers to the ankle and means that it bends inward. When the ankle inverts, the foot supinates.

Got that?
While we're at it, let's mention that pronation has a bad reputation that it doesn't deserve. You have to pronate when you walk. It's part of the way your foot works. When your heel

hits the ground, you touch on the outside of your heel, and you're in a relatively stable supinated position. As your weight moves onto your foot, it pronates, which helps absorb the shock. If you don't pronate a little, you have a high arch and an inflexible foot that can cause problems.

Structure of the Leg

Bones:

The drawing shows the bones of the lower limb from a lateral (outside) view. The main leg bone is the shin bone or *tibia.* It's the second-largest bone in the body, next to the *femur.* On top it supports the weight of the femur (and the rest of your body!), and at the bottom it rests squarely on the talus bone of the foot. Along the sides and in back of this bone, thick layers of muscle protect it, but in front only skin stands between it and the elements. That's why it's so painful to bang your shin into something— there's no muscle to absorb the blow.

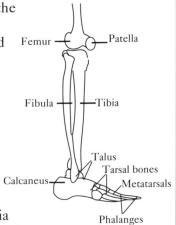

Bones of the lower leg, ankle and foot.

The *fibula* lies next to the tibia on the outside of your lower leg. There's no bone on top of this one and no bone that it really rests on at the bottom. So what's it for?

Together, the tibia and fibula are nature's answer to the I-beam. All along their length, a tough fibrous tissue called the *interosseous membrane* ("inter" meaning between, and "osseus" meaning bone) connects the two bones. This membrane transmits some of the weight from the tibia to the fibula, which acts as a reinforcing unit.

This clever reinforcing act means that both the tibia and fibula can be smaller than the femur on top. The smaller size makes them more flexible and less likely to break. Think of how a thin tree branch will bend, while a thick branch will remain stiff or splinter.

Smaller size also makes the tibia and fibula lighter weight. It would *really* be hard to pull off those aerial flips if you had a femur in your calf! (Remember that stuff about levers and inertia? See Body Basics.)

Isn't it extraordinary how nature planned all this so you could do gymnastics?

Muscles:

Muscles in the leg sit in one of three compartments, separated by thick membranes.

The muscles responsible for dorsal flexion and toe extension sit in the front compartment. They are the *anterior tibialis* (predictably, it's a takeoff of the bone name) and two toe extensor muscles with long names you don't need to know.

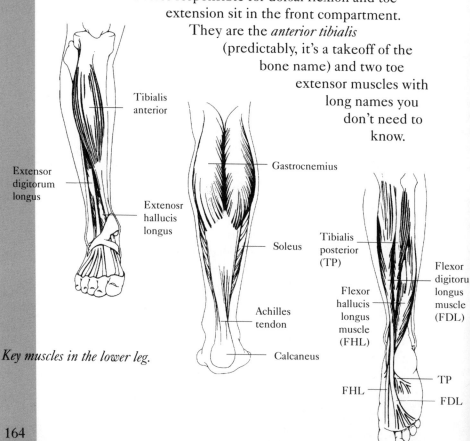

Key muscles in the lower leg.

Moving on to other muscles in the leg: The back muscle compartment contains the calf muscles: the *soleus* (deep layer) and the *gastrocnemius* (surface layer). Soleus comes from the Latin word *solea*, meaning sole, a reference to the shape of the muscle. Gastrocnemius comes from the Greek words *gaster*, meaning stomach, and *kneme*, meaning leg. Maybe the person naming this muscle thought it looked like a stomach. Or maybe he was tired of naming muscles and had all he could stomach. Got any ideas?

Anyway, these two muscles are the ones that enable you to stand up on your toes. The calf muscles make a big contribution in your ability to jump.

Even deeper in the rear muscle compartment are the muscles that stabilize the inside of your ankle to prevent excessive eversion. Lotta long names, so we'll spare you.

The third muscle compartment is a small one on the outside of the fibula. It holds two muscles that stabilize the outside of your ankle and prevent excessive inversion.

Structure of the Ankle

Bones:

What you call the "ankle bones," those bumps that stick out to the side, are really the lower part of the two leg bones. As the front-view drawing shows, these two bumps (the *medial* and *lateral malleolus*) make a sort of protective cap around the dome of the talus bone.

This joint is like a cross between a ball-and-socket joint and a hinge joint, and it offers some of the benefits of both: more stability than the shallow ball-and-socket shoulder joint, and more freedom of motion than a straight hinge joint.

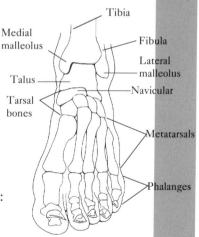

The bones of the ankle and foot.

165

At the beginning of this chapter, we mentioned the design of the talus. If you look at the drawing, you can see that the talus is most narrow under the tibia and widest towards the toes. If you flex your foot, the wide part comes up under the tibia, so you can't move it as far side to side. If you point your toes, you have more room to move sideways. Trivia bit #468.

Ligaments:

Three sets of ligaments connect and stabilize the bones of the ankle joint: the *medial ligament* on the inside, the *lateral ligaments* on the outside, and the *tibiofibular syndesmosis*, a complicated bunch of fibers that hold the tibia and fibula together just above the ankle. The one you're most likely to sprain are the lateral ligaments.

Structure of the Foot

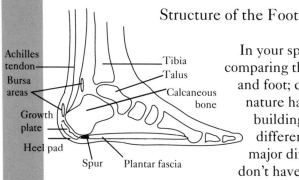

Achilles tendon

Bursa areas

Growth plate

Heel pad

Spur   Plantar fascia

Tibia

Talus

Calcaneous bone

Structure of the foot.

In your spare(!) time, try comparing the bones of the hand and foot; check out the ways nature has used the same basic building blocks for two entirely different functions! One major difference is that humans don't have an opposable big toe to match the thumb. This is where the apes out-do us.

Bones:

The previous drawing on page 165 shows most of the bones in the foot, except for the *calcaneus*, or heel bone. That's easier to see in this side view.

Ligaments, muscles and tendons:

The spring in your step comes partly from the arch of the foot. As you can see in the drawing, your weight falls on your heel and the heads of the metatarsal bones. Both ligaments and muscles help hold this arch in place. Ligaments (not shown) connect the heel bone to the talus and navicular, and the *plantar fascia* muscle on the sole of your foot connects the heel to the metatarsal heads. The plantar fascia is the bowstring for your foot's bony bow.

The whole arrangement is a clever and effective way to absorb shock—that's one reason humans can run long distances without jarring their bodies to rubble. Apes by comparison have very flat feet and would probably not make it through a 10K, much less a marathon.

The *Achilles tendon* connects the heel to the calf muscles and is one of the strongest tendons in the body. In Greek mythology, Achilles was the most heroic of the Greeks who fought in the Trojan War. His mother dipped him in the River Styx when he was an infant, which made every part of his body invulnerable except the heel by which she held him. After impressive heroics in the Trojan War, Achilles was finally brought down by the indignity of a heel wound. A lesson to us all.

COMMON GYMNASTICS INJURIES

Stress Fractures in the Leg

Causes:

Stress fractures of the tibia and fibula frequently result from overuse. When muscles grow tired, they can no longer absorb shock as well. The bones suffer greater stress and may develop hairline cracks along the stress lines. If you don't allow time for healing to take place, the fracture can progress to a full break.

The tibia is the bone most likely to fracture, although the fibula can fracture in sports that require constant muscle tension, like kicking, running and gymnastics.

The chapter on Body Basics shows an x-ray of this type of stress fracture.

Symptoms:

Stress fractures usually begin with mild discomfort. With continued activity, the pain becomes more persistent, lasting from one day to the next. Finally, it hurts too much to go on.

Diagnosis:

X-rays generally don't show stress fractures when they first occur, but only two to four weeks later, if then. The best diagnostic tool is a bone scan.

Treatment:

The cure is rest, changing the training program and correcting any mechanical abnormalities in the foot or gait that may have contributed to the problem. One problem is that gymnasts don't wear shoes, so it is difficult to craft an orthotic solution to the problem. We recommend that you try to work out in shoes with orthotic supports as much as possible. Sometimes arch supports or heel pads in ballet shoes will do the trick. Also, practice your landings in the pit, rather than on mats. When you do use mats, some data suggests that the better the mats are, the fewer the injuries.

Total rest is not necessary for a stress fracture to heal, but the stress must be reduced. You can maintain aerobic conditioning by swimming or cycling instead of running.

It is best to be completely free of symptoms before you start hard workouts on the leg again. However, you can practice and compete with stress fractures under certain circumstances if your doctor approves.

Tibial stress fractures take from six weeks to four months to heal. Fibular fractures usually heal in less than two months because the fibula bears only about ten percent of the body's weight.

Achilles Tendinitis

Cause:

Repetitive overextension or overuse of the Achilles tendon can inflame and thicken the sheath of the tendon. This results in chronic pain and tightness. You are more likely to get this if your calf muscles are very tight, so calf stretching is a good preventive measure.

Symptoms:

The main symptom is pain during workout or after any stretching of the tendon.

Treatment:

Rest the leg and use ice until acute inflammation goes away. To decrease tension on the injured tendon, use a heel lift in your shoes. Once the acute symptoms go away, stretch and strengthen your calf muscles. Use the calf stretch shown in the chapter on Training. Build strength by rising slowly up on your toes and back down again and increasing the repetitions of this exercise.

Ankle Sprains

If you sprain your ankle, you're most likely to sprain the lateral ligaments on the outside of your foot. Sprains to the medial ligaments inside are potentially more dangerous, as they often come along with a fracture of the *lateral malleolus* (outside anklebone), in which case the whole thing may require surgery. Fortunately, medial ligament sprains are not too common.

Causes:

Sprains can happen when the ankle twists inward (spraining the lateral ligaments) or outward (spraining the medial ligaments). They may be mild to severe.

Symptoms:

Sprains cause pain and local swelling. If the damage is great, your ankle may not be stable but tend to slip from side to side.

Diagnosis:

Pain and swelling with a normal x-ray indicate a sprain. Severe sprains may mimic fractures, so you should check with your doctor.

Treatment:

A classic case for RICE in the acute phase. Apply ice immediately, and compress the area with an elastic bandage, taping, or compression pump. Depending on the severity, the ankle may be splinted or braced. Take an anti-inflammatory medication. Follow the directions in the Body Basics chapter.

In two to seven days (after the acute stage) keep the ankle taped but start range-of-motion exercises: gentle ankle rolls. Go swimming or biking to maintain your aerobic fitness and to give the ankle some gentle exercise. Also do contrast soaks two or three times a day: hot water for five minutes followed by cold water for three minutes, repeated twice.

As pain diminishes, build your stretching and conditioning exercises to regain strength in the ankle. There are a number of ways to do this. Perhaps the easiest is to wear a weight boot (or strap a weight to your forefoot) and to do repetitive inversions and eversions, increasing the number of repetitions each day.

The easy way to do inversion is to sit with one leg crossed, injured ankle just past the other knee. Then raise the toes of the injured foot upwards.

For eversion, lie on a bed with your foot hanging over the edge, outer side up. Work against the weight on your foot as you move your foot up and down.

Strengthen other ligaments by slowly rising to your toes and back down. Repeat.

Plantar Fasciitis and Heel Contusions

Causes:

Gymnasts frequently bruise their heels because they spend so much time barefoot. When you work out outside the gym, we recommend that you use good athletic shoes as much as possible. There is no reason that aerobic jogging and similar conditioning work should be done barefoot. It addition, if you're not specifically practicing landings, use the pit. Keep your landings as soft as possible, as often as possible.

Plantar fasciitis is an inflammation of the plantar fascia on the bottom of the foot, caused by (you guessed it) overuse, particularly from hard landings. Remember how the arch of your foot absorbs shock? Well, nature designed it to absorb the shock of walking, not jumping down from ten feet or so. Too many hard landings in a row really dish it out to the poor plantar.

Symptoms:

Heel bruises cause pain in the heel, like a stone bruise. Every step can be torture if it gets bad. This injury happens quickly, unlike plantar fasciitis, which generally creeps up on you.

Plantar fasciitis also causes heel pain, but often the pain will spread along the underside of the foot. If you ignore plantar fasciitis and it becomes chronic, you can get a bone spur on the bottom of the heel. Bone spurs usually arise in older people.

Treatment:

Use ice and massage alternately on the tender area (as described in the previous chapter) and take anti-inflammatory medications. Stretch and exercise in the morning to help loosen up the area before you start stressing it. Stretches include the calf stretch, ankle rolls, and the towel stretch. For the towel stretch, sit on the floor with your foot extended, wrap a towel around the ball of the foot and toes and pull gently for five seconds. Repeat.

For exercises, do toe curls (stand on a towel and use your toes to scrunch it up) and foot rolls (sit down and roll your foot over a tennis ball to massage the plantar muscle).

Sever's Disease

Causes:

Like Osgood-Schlatter's disease, Sever's disease is a growth-plate problem. Sever's is an overuse condition where the growth plate at the end of the *calcaneus* (see the previous drawing) begins to fragment. In some cases, the growth plate can actually pull off, as the *tibial tubercle* can in the knee.

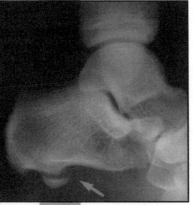

Symptoms:

This problem may mimic Achilles tendinitis, so if you have constant pain at the back of your heel, you should see your doctor. An x-ray of Sever's disease shows the growth plate much whiter than the rest of the calcaneus.

Treatment:

The treatment for Sever's is much like the treatment for Achilles tendinitis.

Avulsion of the growth plate on the calcaneus. This x-ray shows how the growth plate has pulled loose from the rest of the heel bone.

TROUBLESHOOTING: A "DIAGNOSIS" CHART

Here is the ever-present quick reference guide. Please don't
use this chart instead of checking with your doctor!

Troubleshooting your leg,
ankle and foot.

Symptoms and Diagnosis	Acute pain	Chronic or recurring pain	Acute swelling	Late Swelling	Positive X-ray	Positive bone scan
Stress fractures in leg		✓			✓	✓
Achilles tendinitis		✓				
Ankle sprain	✓		✓	✓		
Plantar fasciitis		✓				
Heel contusion	✓			✓		
Sever's disease		✓			✓	✓

SUMMARY

The leg, ankle and foot take an enormous beating in almost any kind of sport and normally do it with incredible aplomb. Gymnastics is particularly hard on your feet because its a sport you have to do barefoot, without technological help. The main advice we have is to use good athletic shoes whenever possible, practice as many landings as possible in the pit, and check with your trainer or doctor at the slightest sign of injury.

Epilogue

It's been fun, but here's the end. You've learned something about your body, something about using it in gymnastics, and something about how to keep it healthy for the long life in front of you.

We hope you feel proud to be the owner of a genuine human body. It's an honor reserved for very few living creatures. You are in charge of an original one-and-only: your own special version of this world's most intricate and wondrous creation. Treasure it.

But what about winning? We titled this book "A Healthy 10"—we've talked about "healthy," but what about the "10?"

People write whole books about winning psychology, but we think it all comes down to three key principles:

Set the right goals.

Contrary to what you might think, winning a gold medal at the Olympics is not the right goal. Why? Two reasons. First, your chances are slim. Think of all the athletes crowding the stadium in Barcelona recently. Only a few came away with gold. And how many never made it to Barcelona? Do you want to spend years honing your gymnastic skills only to end up saying, "Well, I guess that's been ten years down the drain?"

Second, the goal of winning a medal *limits your possibilities*. How many people are able to repeat their performance at the Olympics? Carl Lewis and Mark Spitz are the exceptions. Nearly everyone who peaks with a gold medal limits their future accomplishments. Having achieved the "ultimate goal," they are unable to do it again.

Winning football teams play right on through the goal posts, as if the field went on forever. The quarterback passes

176

deep into the end zone, not to the one-yard line. Losers stall out, over-awed by the nearness of those white posts.

So what is the right goal? Simple. *To be as much yourself as you can be.* To do what you can do, as well as you can do it. To express yourself as fully as possible, every minute. Don't dwell on the mistakes of the past. Don't worry about the future.

To be a real winner, your goal should be to live—and enjoy—every moment to its fullest. From the simplest training to the most demanding meet.

Rehearse mentally.

Gymnastics is as much in your mind as your body. Close your eyes and visualize some difficult maneuver. . .Do you have a vision of every move you make? Can you actually feel your body making the move? Do you know where you are in the air, what every part of your body is doing? Make a movie in your mind, play it over in slow motion and refine it until it's perfect. Then speed up the projector. . .You'll be amazed how much this adds to your skill. Studies show that athletes can often gain as much or more benefit from mental rehearsal as they do from physical practice.

Make this technique a habit of training. Use mental gymnastics to fall asleep at night—if you dream the perfect move, you won't believe how much that dream will carry over!

And use this technique at meets. Before you start, see yourself doing the routine. See everything happening perfectly and naturally from beginning to end. Then give yourself and your body to this vision.

Epilogue

Focus.

This means living in the "now-ness" of what you are doing—in training and at meets. It means participating fully, without distraction, in every second that you move through.

Focus means that you don't stand mentally to one side, judging your performance. It means that you don't remember that only a few seconds ago you fell off the beam. It means that you don't worry about what the point standings are, or whether the judges are biased. It means that you live fully, *now*. It means living with love for the sport and joy in your skill. It has very little to do with "performing" for some transitory honor.

Enjoy!

The Creator has given each of us unique gifts— perhaps even a real talent for gymnastics. When we use our gifts with love and joy, we celebrate what we have received and we glorify life itself. That's the real "10."

Think about the people you admire most. Remember Mary Lou Retton's smile? She had that "joy of life" and it showed. (The judges saw it too.)

When you enjoy yourself, you literally "lighten up." You fly higher, run faster, and balance more beautifully than you ever thought possible—because it's no longer so terribly important to be perfect.

It's too late to worry about technique when you get to a meet. You know it or you don't. Your body has memorized the moves or not. Worrying poisons your energy, short-circuits your wiring, and sabotages your talent.

A paradox: We achieve perfection when we least seek it.

Work hard, practice your skills, develop your body and take care of it. When the time comes, give your body the freedom to create the beauty it knows, while your mind rejoices in the amazement of this creation. Let go, live in the present and let the numbers take care of themselves! It's a daring technique, and it works. Better than that, it becomes a way of life.

Your journey in this world can be rich with "10" experiences, regardless of what the judges think. Isn't this what really counts?

INDEX

P

Parents 67
Pars interarticularis 102
Patella 120, 121
Pediatrics 5
Phalange 154
Phosphorus 14
Physical medicine 4
Physical therapist 9
Physical therapy 9
Plantar extension 162
Plantar fasciitis 171
Plantar flexion 162
Plyometrics training 75
Posterior cruciate ligament 120
Press handstand 96
Progressive resistance 77
Pronation 162
Proprioception 41
Protein 48, 50
Psychiatrists 10
Psychologists 10
Psychology 175
Puberty 44
Pushups on parallel bars 91

Q

Q-angle 128
Quad stretch 87
Quadriceps wall sit 91

R

Radial head fracture 152
Radial styloid 154
Radius 146

Radius and ulna fractures 156
Rectus abdominus 104
RICE 24
Rotator cuff 139
   tear 140
Rubber bands 81

S

Sacroiliac 19
Sacrum 103
Scaphoid navicular 154
Scaphoid navicular fracture 156
Scapula 137
Scheurmann's disease 113
Scoliosis 107
Scotty-dog fracture 102, 108
Sever's disease 172
Sever's condition 17
Shoulder 137
   bones, ligaments
      and bursae 138
   dislocation 144, 145
   impingement 140
   instability 143, 144
   labrum injuries 145
   structure 138
Shoulder joint 20
Shoulder stretch 87
SIT muscles 139
Skeletal muscles 21
Skeleton 14
Slipped disc 115
Soleus 165
Somatotype 35
Spinal canal 101
Spinal column 103
Spine 99